Strategies, Techniques, & Approaches to Thinking

Critical Thinking Cases in Nursing

FOURTH EDITION

Sandra Luz Martinez de Castillo, EdD, RN

Director of the Nursing Program
Los Medanos College
Pittsburg, California

SAUNDERS
ELSEVIER

SAUNDERS
ELSEVIER

11830 Westline Industrial Drive
St. Louis, MO 63146

STRATEGIES, TECHNIQUES, & APPROACHES TO THINKING:
CRITICAL THINKING CASES IN NURSING

ISBN 978-1-4160-6152-6

Notice

Knowledge and best practice in this field are constantly changing. As new research and experience broaden our knowledge, changes in practice, treatment and drug therapy may become necessary or appropriate. Readers are advised to check the most current information provided (i) on procedures featured or (ii) by the manufacturer of each product to be administered, to verify the recommended dose or formula, the method and duration of administration, and contraindications. It is the responsibility of the practitioner, relying on their own experience and knowledge of the patient, to make diagnoses, to determine dosages and the best treatment for each individual patient, and to take all appropriate safety precautions. To the fullest extent of the law, neither the Publisher nor the Authors assumes any liability for any injury and/or damage to persons or property arising out of or related to any use of the material contained in this book.

The Publisher

ISBN 978-1-4160-6152-6

Senior Editor: Kristin Geen
Developmental Editor: Jamie Horn
Publishing Services Manager: Deborah L. Vogel
Project Manager: Pat Costigan
Book Designer: Charlie Seibel

Printed in Canada

Last digit is the print number: 9 8 7 6 5 4 3 2 1

PREFACE

Dear Nursing Student:

You are using this manual because you have decided to become a nurse! Congratulations, nursing is a wonderful profession. Professional nurses are vital to the practice of nursing. Nursing involves more than knowing how to perform a skill competently. Rather, nursing is feeling passionate about the care you give and genuinely caring for the whole person and the family. As you learn to provide care for the whole person, you will experience nursing in its purest sense.

Learning is so exciting, and now with the use of technology, you can really make your learning interactive. There is a lot to learn in order to be a competent, safe practitioner. An integral part of being a safe practitioner is applying critical thinking skills. Critical thinking is more than problem solving. Critical thinking is a process that requires you to think about or reflect on your decisions, actions, skills, knowledge, attitudes, beliefs, etc., for the purpose of providing safe nursing care. I am sure you use critical thinking every day. However, in nursing practice, your knowledge base and experience will assist you to use critical thinking and apply clinical reasoning to make clinical decisions for individual patient care situations.

The manual is designed to assist you to apply and use critical thinking to common patient care situations. This manual is divided into six sections. **Section One** will help you apply learned knowledge to several short clinical case studies and patient care situations. It is important to focus on how the theoretical concepts and principles assist the nurse to make clinical decisions. The case studies in Section One have dual purposes: (1) to reinforce fundamental concepts and principles and (2) to demonstrate how learned knowledge is applied to patient care situations. Notice how nurses use their knowledge in clinical practice to make decisions. Remember that knowledge is fundamental to critical thinking, so get involved in knowledge building learning activities.

Section Two presents case studies that will help you prioritize and make sound clinical decisions. In the clinical setting, the nurse directs and manages the care of several patients, so Section Two presents progressive case studies that allow you to see how nurses need to constantly make clinical decisions based on patient care situations. It is important to discuss the clinical situation and your decisions and rationales with your peers and your instructor. The discussion process provides an opportunity to hear other points of view and rationales that may need to be considered before making the clinical decision. The nursing process is included in this section to assist you in applying the components of assessment, nursing diagnosis, planning, and implementation.

Section Three presents clinical situations using an intershift report format. The presenting situation is given through the intershift report. Like the intershift report process encountered in the clinical setting, relevant and irrelevant information is presented. You are asked to **analyze** and **interpret** the data based on the presenting situation. Flow charts in the form of the patient's Nursing Care Rand/Kardex, Medication Record, Intake and Output Record, Nursing Notes, and History and Physical are provided to assist you in gathering further data. This activity helps you (1) focus on gathering the data, both from the report and the flow charts, and (2) make relevant connections and synthesize the data. All of these activities are part of using critical thinking and clinical reasoning to make patient care decisions.

Section Four focuses on the development of management and leadership skills. As you begin to work with peers and to delegate to staff, work-related issues and personnel situations will arise. As with the patient care situations, it is important to apply critical thinking skills to work through the various case studies. As you work through a case study with peers, take a moment to focus on your management and leadership skills. Do you have a preferred style of management or leadership? Further, look at the leadership and management style of the nurses in clinical practice.

Section Five provides additional test questions to assist you in testing your knowledge and to help you apply test-taking strategies.

Section Six offers three situations that continue to assist you in applying your nursing knowledge and enhancing your leadership and delegation skills. In this section, you are introduced to evidence-based practice and encouraged to begin the processes of questioning, exploring, and researching nursing practices. Finally, the concept of caring for the whole person is synthesized in the Caring for the Whole Person diagram. Through the use of this diagram, you will review the fundamental needs of the patient and apply caring and advocacy to support the individual patient or family.

In addition, the following icon ⓔ can be found on selected case studies. This icon indicates that additional information can be accessed at the Evolve website at *http://evolve.elsevier.com/castillo/thinking*. For example, in Section One, under the Respiratory case study, after accessing the web link you will hear audible breath sounds, and under the Skin Integrity case study, you will be able to access the Braden Scale in order to complete the case study.

The nursing student is encouraged to use the **Critical Thinking Model** to purposefully work on developing critical thinking skills and make decisions based on clinical reasoning. Your instructor will ask you many questions that will assist you to use your knowledge and help you to apply critical thinking skills in clinical practice. I hope you enjoy learning from these case studies.

DEDICATION

Para mi papa—amor de mis amores
Que alegría cuando uno llega a realizar su deseo (02-07-08)

REVIEWERS

Debi Beitler, RN, MSN, FNP
Instructor
Associate Degree Program
Long Beach City College
Long Beach, California

Aaron Buck, MSN, RN, CPNP
Assistant Dean of Nursing/Assistant Professor
Chamberlain College of Nursing
St. Louis, Missouri

Michele Cislo, RN, MA, CPN
Associate Professor
Practical Nursing
Union County College
Plainfield, New Jersey

Mary A. Gers, MSN, CNS, RNC
Associate Professor
School of Nursing and Health Professions
Northern Kentucky University
Highland Heights, Kentucky

Sherry Goertz
Nursing Faculty
College of Health and Human Development,
School of Nursing
The Pennsylvania State University
Mont Alto, Pennsylvania

Susan A. Sandstrom, MSN, RN, BC, CNE
Associate Professor in Nursing
School of Health Professions
College of Saint Mary
Omaha, Nebraska

Katherine Seibert, MEd, RN
Associate Professor of Nursing
Mercy College of Health Sciences
Des Moines, Iowa

Beryl Stetson, RNBC, MSN
Assistant Professor - Nursing
Health Science Education Department
Raritan Valley Community College
Somerville, New Jersey

ACKNOWLEDGMENT

To all my students—who continue to foster
my joy of teaching . . .
To Jamie Horn and Pat Costigan from Elsevier. Thank you for your
patience and assistance with this edition.

CONTENTS

Section One—Cognitive-Building Critical Thinking Activities

Section Two—Priority-Setting and Decision-Making Activities

Section One - Cognitive-Building Critical Thinking Activities

PROFESSIONAL NURSING PRACTICE

Fill in the blanks with the requested information:

PATIENT SAFETY

List the function(s) of the Boards of Registered Nursing or the Professional Regulatory Body

- ______________________________
- ______________________________
- ______________________________
- ______________________________
- ______________________________

Identify the professional nurses associations that influence nursing practice:

-
-
-
-
-

Basis for the scope of nursing practice

-
-
-
-
-
-

Case Study: A student nurse started clinical practice in the acute care setting. The assignment includes caring for a client who will be transferred to a skilled facility today but needs morning care, bathing, and assistance with feeding before discharge. The client also has an indwelling urinary catheter.

Pertinent Terminology	Definition
Nurse Practice Act	
Scope of nursing practice	
Independent nursing functions	
Dependent nursing functions	
Interdependent nursing functions	

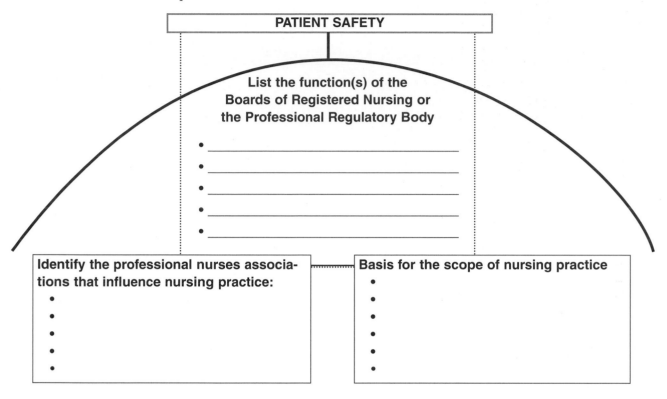

From the case study, identify the type of nursing function for the following interventions:

Assigned Nursing Care	Function
Morning care, bathing, feeding, indwelling urinary catheter care	☐ Independent ☐ Dependent ☐ Interdependent

The family arrives and asks whether the father will be transferred to the skilled facility with the urinary catheter. The student consults with the RN, who says that "it should probably be removed."

Assigned Nursing Care	Assigned Nursing Care
Urinary catheter removal	☐ Independent ☐ Dependent ☐ Interdependent

The RN and the student return to the client's room. The RN is getting ready to administer the morning medications to the client.

Assigned Nursing Care	Assigned Nursing Care
Administration of medication	☐ Independent ☐ Dependent ☐ Interdependent

Interactive Activity: With a partner, connect to the website of the Board of Registered Nursing or the professional regulatory body for your state and review the regulations governing the scope of practice for the following situations.

1. What is the position of the State Board of Registered Nursing or the professional regulatory body of the state regarding services provided by student nurses?

2. What is the position of the State Board of Registered Nursing or the professional regulatory body of the state regarding delegation of tasks?

VITAL SIGNS

List the routes for taking a **temperature**:

1. ______________________________
2. ______________________________
3. ______________________________
4. ______________________________

The **blood pressure** may be auscultated in the

________________ and ________________ spaces.

Use the diagram to identify the **pulse sites** in the body.

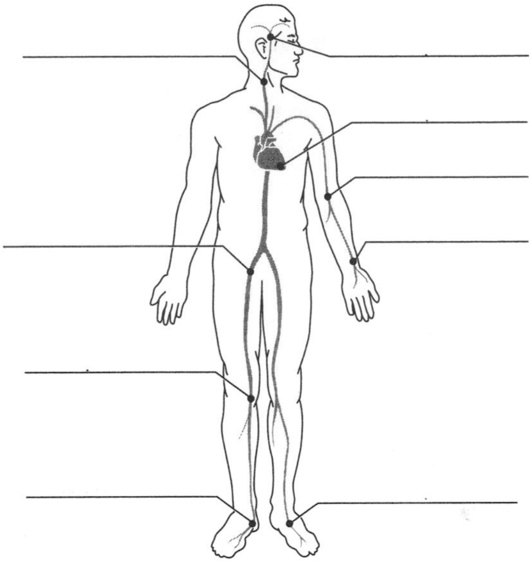

Case Study: An adult male client has been having a high fever for 2 days. At the physician's office he was found to be febrile. Additionally, the client is complaining of chills, night sweats, anorexia, and fatigue. He is admitted to the hospital. The physician's orders include vital signs (VS) every 4 hours. On admission he had pyrexia. The admission VS are T 102.4° F, P 96, R 26, BP 148/88.

Pertinent Terminology	Definition
Vital signs	______________________________
Temperature	______________________________
Pulse	______________________________
Respiration	______________________________
Blood pressure	______________________________
Febrile	______________________________
Pyrexia	______________________________
Anorexia	______________________________
Fatigue	______________________________

From the case study, record today's date and the admission VS on the **Graphic Sheet** below. Enter the following vital signs for today:

1200	T 103.6° F,	P 108,	R 32,	BP 160/76
1600	T 101.2° F,	P 98,	R 28,	BP 154/82
2000	T 100.0° F,	P 80,	R 24,	BP 150/90

Record the 0800 VS for the next day: T 99.6° F, P 72, R 18, BP 146/94

Draw a line between the temperature recordings to create a graph.

Graphic Sheet

Date												
Time	0400	0800	1200	1600	2000	2400	0400	0800	1200	1600	2000	2400
40° C 104° F												
39.4° C 103° F												
38.9° C 102° F												
38.3° C 101° F												
37.7° C 100° F												
37.2° C 99° F												
37 36.6° C 98° F												
36.1° C 97° F												
35.5° C 96° F												
Pulse												
Resp.												
BP												

Interactive Activity: With a partner, identify the **normal range(s)** for the VS in the adult.

Body temperature **Oral** ____________________

Axillary ____________________

Rectal ____________________

Pulse ________________

Respirations ________________

Blood Pressure ________________

TEMPERATURE

The **body temperature** is regulated through the

_________________________.

Body temperature is affected by:

1. ______________________________
2. ______________________________
3. ______________________________
4. ______________________________
5. ______________________________
6. ______________________________

Body temperature remains constant through **heat production** and **heat loss**.

Factors that influence heat production:

- ______________________________
- ______________________________

Factors that influence heat loss:

- ______________________________
- ______________________________
- ______________________________
- ______________________________

Case Study: A 79-year-old client was brought to the emergency department after having been found unconscious at home. The physician has admitted the client with the diagnosis of heat stroke. On admission the vital signs are: T 40.5° C, P 100, R 16, BP 118/64. The client's skin is flushed and feels hot and dry. The client is now alert and complaining of nausea. The physician orders the temperature to be monitored every hour.

Pertinent Terminology	Definition
Temperature	
Hyperthermia	
Hypothermia	
Heat stroke	
Conduction	
Convection	
Evaporation	
Radiation	

From the case study, explain how the **evaporation factor** contributed to the client's development of heat stroke:

Fill in the thermometers to reflect the temperature readings (both Celsius and Fahrenheit) for your shift.

Time	Reading
0900	- 39.8° C
1000	- 40.1° C
1100	- 38.7° C
1200	- 103.8° F
1300	- 102.6° F
1400	- 101.4° F
1500	- 100.2° F

Non-mercury Thermometer

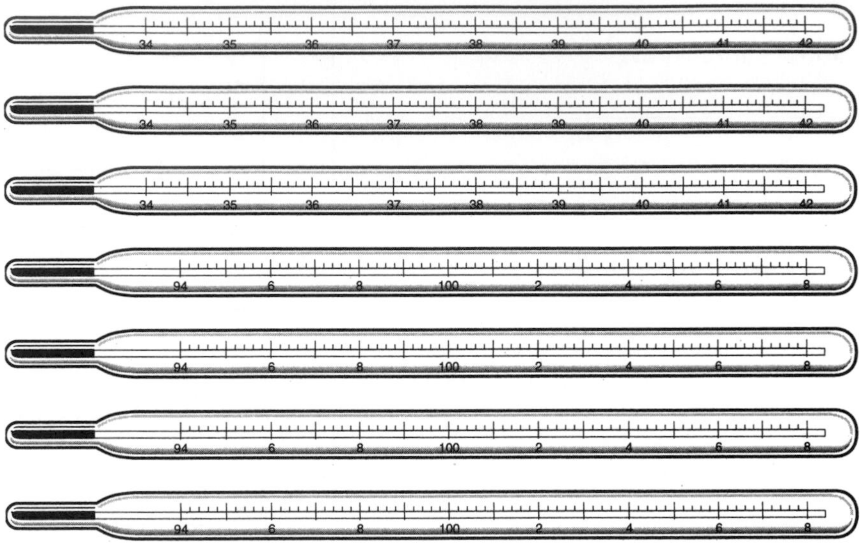

Interactive Activity: **Graph** the temperature readings for your shift. Draw a line between each temperature recording. Compare your **Temperature Recording Sheet** with that of a partner.

Temperature Recording Sheet

Time	0800	0900	1000	1100	1200	1300	1400	1500
40.5° C 105° F								
40° C 104° F								
39.4° C 103° F								
38.9° C 102° F								
38.3° C 101° F								
37.7° C 100° F								
37.2° C 99° F								
37 **36.6° C** 98° F								
36.1° C 97° F								
35.5° C 96° F								

APPLYING CRITICAL THINKING SKILLS TO TEST QUESTIONS

INSTRUCTIONS: Circle the one best answer for each test question. Write your rationale for selecting the answer. To enhance your learning and test-taking skills, discuss your answer and rationale with a partner. The answer and the rationale can be found on the back of this page.

1. The nurse is using a digital thermometer to take an oral temperature. After taking the oral temperature, the nurse obtains a reading of 94.2° F. Which follow-up action is most appropriate for the nurse to do?
   a. Use another digital thermometer to retake the temperature.
   b. Feel the client's skin temperature.
   c. Take a rectal temperature.
   d. Document the findings.

   Rationale for your selection: ______________________________

2. The nurse obtains an axillary temperature of 97.4° F on a client. In graphing the temperature, it is most appropriate for the nurse to:
   a. write "see nurse's notes" above the temperature reading.
   b. identify the temperature reading with an "Ax."
   c. graph the oral equivalent temperature of 98.4° F.
   d. just graph 97.4° F on the form.

   Rationale for your selection: ______________________________

3. The nurse is caring for a client who has an oral temperature of 99.6° F at 8:00 AM, the start of the day shift. The client's Kardex indicates that vitals signs should be taken once a shift. In planning care for the client, which action is most appropriate?
   a. Ensure that the temperature is taken promptly at 4:00 PM.
   b. Call the physician for a more frequent order.
   c. Take the temperature as necessary.
   d. Begin cooling measures.

   Rationale for your selection: ______________________________

ANSWER KEY FOR APPLYING CRITICAL THINKING SKILLS TO TEST QUESTIONS

HELPFUL HINTS: Read all test questions carefully. Identify key words in the question that will guide you in answering the question. In these test questions the **key words** to consider are **"follow-up"** and **"most appropriate."** Compare your rationale with the one in the test question.

1. The nurse is using a digital thermometer to take an oral temperature. After taking the oral temperature, the nurse obtains a reading of 94.2° F. Which follow-up action is most appropriate for the nurse to do?
   (a.) Use another digital thermometer to retake the temperature.
   b. Feel the client's skin temperature.
   c. Take a rectal temperature.
   d. Document the findings.

   Rationale: The answer is (a). Because the nurse is using a digital thermometer, it is important for the nurse to ensure that the equipment is functioning. The temperature recording is low and should be taken again. Options (b) and (c) are not appropriate; option (d) should be done after the temperature is verified.

2. The nurse obtains an axillary temperature of 97.4° F on a client. In graphing the temperature, it is most appropriate for the nurse to:
   a. write "see nurse's notes" above the temperature reading.
   (b.) identify the temperature reading with an "Ax."
   c. graph the oral equivalent temperature of 98.4° F.
   d. just graph 97.4° F on the form.

   Rationale: The answer is (b). It is important for the nurse to identify the appropriate information on where the temperature was taken. Options (a), (c), and (d) do not accurately document the temperature information.

3. The nurse is caring for a client who has an oral temperature of 99.6° F at 8:00 AM, the start of the day shift. The client's Kardex indicates that vitals signs should be taken once a shift. In planning care for the client, which action is most appropriate?
   a. Ensure that the temperature is taken promptly at 4:00 PM.
   b. Call the physician for a more frequent order.
   (c.) Take the temperature as necessary.
   d. Begin cooling measures.

   Rationale: The answer is (c). The nurse can make an independent decision to take the temperature more frequently to ensure safe nursing care. Option (a) does not allow for a thorough, ongoing assessment. Options (b) and (d) are not necessary at this time.

PULSE

The normal **pulse rate range** for an adult is:

____

The **pulse characteristics** includes a description of the _____________, _____________, and _________________________ of the pulse.

The **pulse** is affected by:

1. ___________________________
2. ___________________________
3. ___________________________
4. ___________________________
5. ___________________________
6. ___________________________
7. ___________________________
8. ___________________________

Draw circles on the diagram that identify the sites where the **pulse** is found in the body.

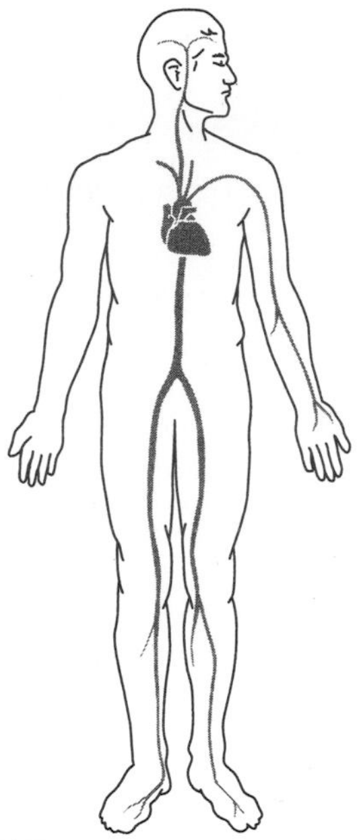

Case Study: A 52-year-old male client has been complaining of a rapid heartbeat. He says that it feels as if his "heart is racing." His wife took him to the urgent care clinic where he was found to have an irregular pulse of 160 bpm; he was transferred to the hospital. On admission to the hospital his vital signs are T 98.4° F, P 168, R 28, BP 146/90. His skin is moist and he is very anxious. The physician orders the administration of cardiac medications and for the pulse to be monitored every 2 hours.

Pertinent Terminology	Definition
Pulse	______________________
Peripheral pulse	______________________
Apical pulse	______________________
Stroke volume	______________________
Cardiac output	______________________
Pulse rhythm	______________________
Pulse quality	______________________
Tachycardia	______________________
Bradycardia	______________________
Arrhythmia	______________________
Pulse deficit	______________________

From the case study, use the admission pulse of 168 bpm to assist in identifying the words in the parentheses that would **best describe** the characteristics of this pulse:

Pulse Characteristic	Descriptive Words	Selected Word(s)
Rate	(rapid, tachycardia, bradycardia, increased)	________________
Rhythm	(regular, irregular, abnormal, dysrhythmia)	________________
Quality	(weak, thready, bounding, difficult to palpate)	________________

Interactive Activity: With a partner, identify the **pulse site** in each diagram and **write in the reason** for checking the pulse from this area.

Pulse: ________________

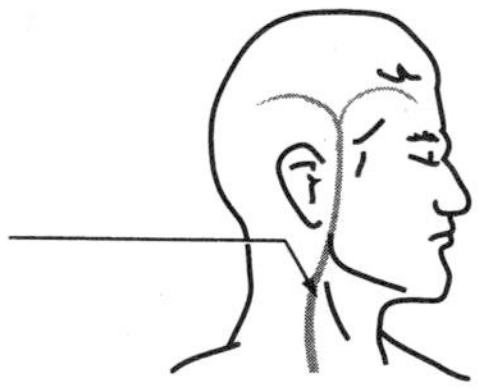

Reason: ________________

Pulse: ________________

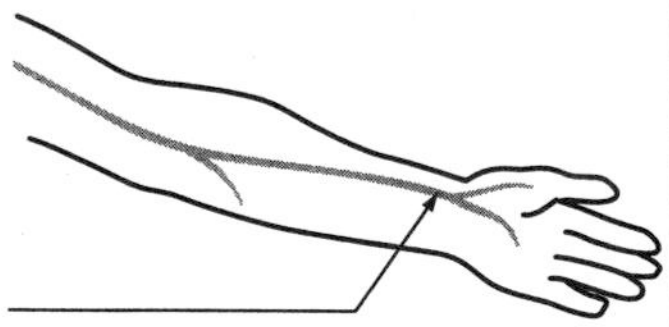

Reason: ________________

Pulse: ________________

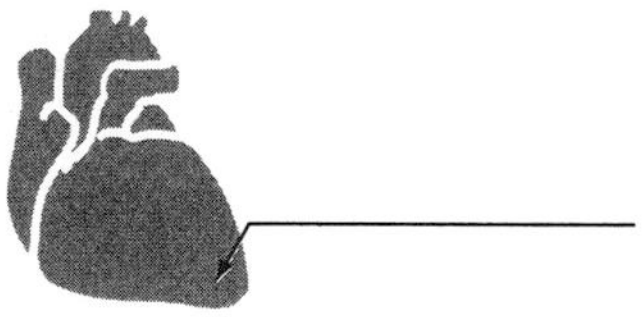

Reason: ________________

Pulse: ________________

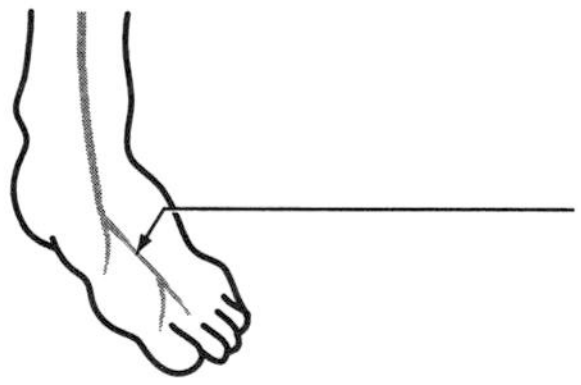

Reason: ________________

The **apical pulse** is taken when ________________________________.

To take an **apical pulse**, the stethoscope is placed on ________________________________.

APPLYING CRITICAL THINKING SKILLS TO TEST QUESTIONS

INSTRUCTIONS: **Circle the one best answer for each test question.** Write your rationale for selecting the answer. To enhance your learning and test-taking skills, discuss your answer and rationale with a partner. The answer and the rationale can be found on the back of this page.

1. The nurse describes the radial pulse as "thready and irregular" after taking morning vital signs. The most appropriate follow-up nursing action is to:
   a. notify the physician.
   b. check the apical pulse.
   c. graph the pulse.
   d. check the previous pulse.

   Rationale for your selection: ______________________________
   ____
   ____
   ____
   ____
   ____

2. The nurse is auscultating an apical pulse on a client. In counting the apical pulse, the nurse counts:
   a. each lub-dub as one beat.
   b. each lub-dub as two beats.
   c. the pulse for 10 seconds and multiplies by 6.
   d. the pulse for 30 seconds and multiplies by 2.

   Rationale for your selection: ______________________________
   ____
   ____
   ____
   ____
   ____

3. The nurse is instructed to check for a pedal pulse on a client at the beginning of the shift. To carry out this intervention, it is most appropriate for the nurse to:
   a. count the brachial pulse for 30 seconds.
   b. count the posterior tibial pulse for 1 full minute.
   c. palpate for the dorsalis pedis.
   d. palpate for the popliteal pulse.

   Rationale for your selection: ______________________________
   ____
   ____
   ____
   ____
   ____

ANSWER KEY FOR APPLYING CRITICAL THINKING SKILLS TO TEST QUESTIONS

HELPFUL HINTS: Read all test questions carefully. Identify key words in the question that will guide you in answering the question. In these test questions the **key words** to consider are **"most appropriate."** Compare your rationale with the one in the test question.

1. The nurse describes the radial pulse as "thready and irregular" after taking morning vital signs. The most appropriate follow-up nursing action is to:
   a. notify the physician.
   (b.) check the apical pulse.
   c. graph the pulse.
   d. check the previous pulse.

   Rationale: The answer is (b). It is the nurse's responsibility to validate abnormal findings. Therefore, the most appropriate follow-up action in this question is to check the apical pulse. This will assist the nurse to fully assess the findings. Although options (a), (c), and (d) are actions that the nurse would do, they are not the most appropriate for this situation.

2. The nurse is auscultating an apical pulse on a client. In counting the apical pulse, the nurse counts:
   (a.) each lub-dub as one beat.
   b. each lub-dub as two beats.
   c. the pulse for 10 seconds and multiplies by 6.
   d. the pulse for 30 seconds and multiplies by 2.

   Rationale: The answer is (a). Each lub represents the closure of the mitral and tricuspid valves during systole and the dub represents the closure of the aortic and pulmonic valves during diastole. Together the lub-dub sounds are counted as one beat. Options (b), (c), and (d) do not describe the correct technique for counting the apical pulse.

3. The nurse is instructed to check for a pedal pulse on a client at the beginning of the shift. To carry out this intervention, it is most appropriate for the nurse to:
   a. count the brachial pulse for 30 seconds.
   b. count the posterior tibial pulse for 1 full minute.
   (c.) palpate for the dorsalis pedis.
   d. palpate for the popliteal pulse.

   Rationale: The answer is (c). This question addresses the nurse's understanding of pedal pulses. Therefore, in this situation, it is most appropriate for the nurse to locate and palpate the pulse in the feet. Although option (b) identifies one of the pedal pulses, it is not necessary to take a pedal pulse for a full minute. Options (a) and (d) are not appropriate in carrying out this nursing order.

RESPIRATION

The normal **respiration rate range** for an adult is ________________.

The **characteristics of respiration** include a description of the __________, __________, and __________ of the respirations.

The factors that affect the **characteristics of the respiration** include:

1. ______________________________
2. ______________________________
3. ______________________________
4. ______________________________
5. ______________________________
6. ______________________________
7. ______________________________
8. ______________________________
9. ______________________________

A **normal** respiratory pattern consists of a full inspiration and a full expiration counted over one minute as the diagram illustrates:

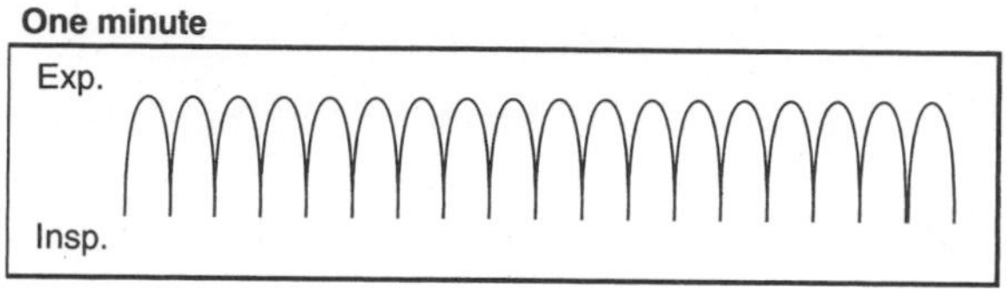

The diagram demonstrates a ______________ respiratory pattern.

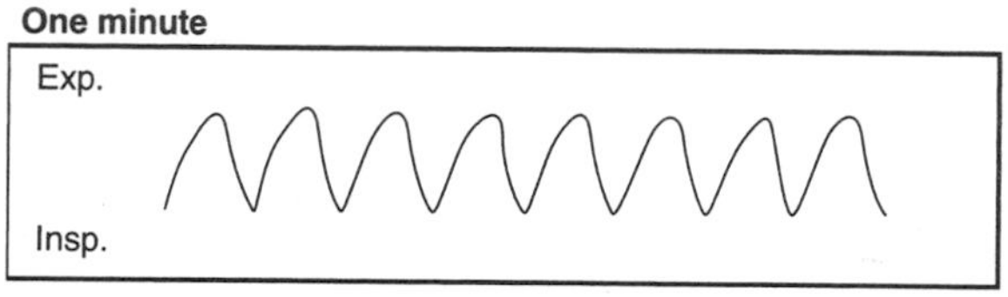

The diagram demonstrates a ______________ respiratory pattern.

Case Study: A male client has been a smoker for 20 years. He has noticed increased shortness of breath (SOB) for the past 6 months and is complaining of a productive cough with thick whitish phlegm. The nurse notices that his respiratory rate is 32 and regular and describes his lung sounds as fine crackling sounds heard on inspiration. Pulse oximetry is 92% on room air.

Pertinent Terminology	Definition
Respiration	
Tachypnea	
Bradypnea	
Eupnea	
Apnea	
Orthopnea	
Dyspnea	
Cheyne-Stokes	
Kussmaul	
Phlegm	
Pulse oximetry	

From the case study, use the respiratory rate of 32 to assist in identifying the words in the parentheses that would **best describe** the characteristics of this respiratory pattern:

Respiratory Characteristic	Descriptive Words	Selected Word(s)
Rate	(eupnea, tachypnea, bradypnea, apnea)	______________
Depth	(deep, full inspiration/expiration, short, shallow)	______________
Rhythm	(regular, irregular)	______________

Draw a line to match the **identified lung sounds** below with the appropriate description. (Visit *http://evolve.elsevier.com/castillo/thinking* to hear sample lung sounds.)

Wheeze	crackling sound, may be fine or coarse, heard frequently on inspiration
Crackle	coarse, harsh, loud sound, best heard on expiration
Rhonchi	continuous high-pitched musical sound best heard on expiration

Circle the lung sound that best describes the client's lung sounds.

Interactive Activity: Draw a diagram that represents the respiratory pattern identified under each box. Compare and discuss your diagrams with a partner.

1 minute

Respiration Pattern: ______________

1 minute

Respiration Pattern: ______________

1 minute

Respiration Pattern: ______________

1 minute

Respiration Pattern: ______________

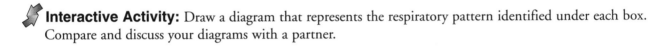

APPLYING CRITICAL THINKING SKILLS TO TEST QUESTIONS

INSTRUCTIONS: Circle the one best answer for each test question. Write your rationale for selecting the answer. To enhance your learning and test-taking skills, discuss your answer and rationale with a partner. The answer and the rationale can be found on the back of this page.

1. The nurse is taking the vital signs of a client who has shortness of breath. In counting the respiratory rate it is most important for the nurse to:
   a. observe the rise and fall of the chest for 15 seconds.
   b. describe the respiratory pattern.
   c. sit the client in a semi-Fowler's position.
   d. count the respiratory rate for 1 minute.

   Rationale for your selection: ____________________

2. The nurse assesses the respiratory rate of an adult client to be 20 and unlabored. The most appropriate follow-up nursing intervention is to:
   a. reassess the respiratory rate.
   b. graph the findings.
   c. check the pulse oximeter.
   d. place the client in high-Fowler's position.

   Rationale for your selection: ____________________

3. The physician orders pulse oximetry checks on the client once a shift. To effectively use the pulse oximeter on the client, the nurse would:
   a. place the pulse oximeter on the client's finger and wait for a reading.
   b. give the client oxygen before using the pulse oximeter.
   c. place the client in high-Fowler's position.
   d. use the pulse oximeter only when the client has dyspnea.

   Rationale for your selection: ____________________

ANSWER KEY FOR APPLYING CRITICAL THINKING SKILLS TO TEST QUESTIONS

HELPFUL HINTS: Read all test questions carefully. Identify key words in the question that will guide you in answering the question. In these test questions the **key words** to consider are **"most important," "most appropriate,"** and **"effectively use."** Compare your rationale with the one found for each question.

1. The nurse is taking the vital signs of a client who has shortness of breath. In counting the respiratory rate it is most important for the nurse to:
   a. observe the rise and fall of the chest for 15 seconds.
   b. describe the respiratory pattern.
   c. sit the client in a semi-Fowler's position.
   (d.) count the respiratory rate for 1 minute.

   Rationale: The answer is (d). Because the client has shortness of breath, it is most important for the nurse to fully assess the respirations for 1 minute. Option (a) does not allow the nurse to fully assess the respiratory pattern; option (b) is good but does not provide a time frame, and option (c) compromises the respiratory system.

2. The nurse assesses the respiratory rate of an adult client to be 20 and unlabored. The most appropriate follow-up nursing intervention is to:
   a. reassess the respiratory rate.
   (b.) graph the findings.
   c. check the pulse oximeter.
   d. place the client in high-Fowler's position.

   Rationale: The answer is (b). The findings are normal; therefore, the next nursing intervention is to graph the findings. Options (a), (c), and (d) can be performed if the nurse assesses an abnormal rate.

3. The physician orders pulse oximetry checks on the client once a shift. To effectively use the pulse oximeter on the client, the nurse would:
   (a.) place the pulse oximeter on the client's finger and wait for a reading.
   b. give the client oxygen before using the pulse oximeter.
   c. place the client in high-Fowler's position.
   d. use the pulse oximeter only when the client has dyspnea.

   Rationale: The answer is (a). The answer describes how to use the pulse oximeter. Options (b) and (c) are incorrect in answering how to effectively use the pulse oximeter. Option (d) is incorrect: a pulse oximeter can be used to assess oxygenation in any client.

BLOOD PRESSURE

The normal blood pressure for an adult is ______________________.

Factors that affect the blood pressure include:

1. ______________________
2. ______________________
3. ______________________
4. ______________________
5. ______________________
6. ______________________
7. ______________________
8. ______________________
9. ______________________
10. ______________________

Identify the parts of the following items used in obtaining a blood pressure:

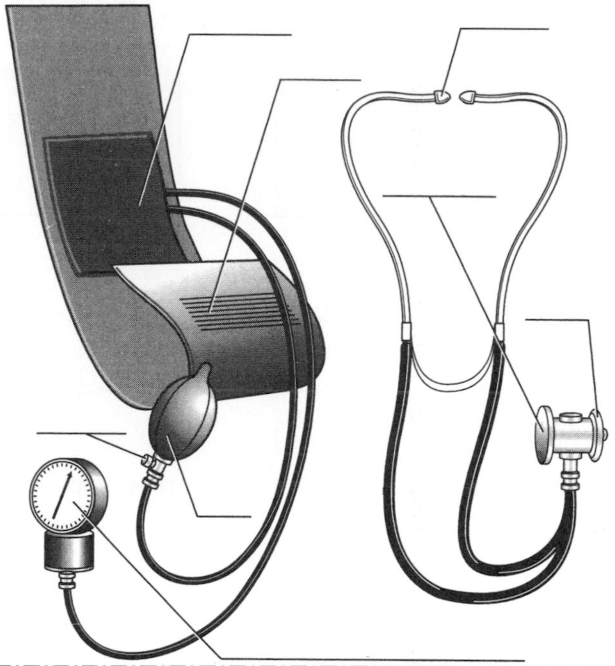

Case Study: A 65-year-old African-American man goes weekly to the hypertension clinic for blood pressure checks. He has a 20-year history of smoking 2 packs of cigarettes a day. His father died from heart disease and his brother has hypertension. His current blood pressure reading is 174/104, and he is complaining of a headache and dizziness when getting up in the morning.

Pertinent Terminology	Definition
Blood pressure	______________________
Systolic pressure	______________________
Diastolic pressure	______________________
Korotkoff's sounds	______________________
Pulse pressure	______________________
Prehypertension	______________________
Hypertension	______________________
Hypotension	______________________
Orthostatic hypotension	______________________
Auscultatory gap	______________________

From the case study, identify the **factors** that predisposed the patient for development of hypertension:

____________________ ____________________ ____________________

____________________ ____________________ ____________________

The clinic nurse monitors the patient's blood pressure for 3 days:

Day 1	
11:00 AM	210/110
11:15 AM	202/104
11:30 AM	190/98

Day 2	
11:00 AM	188/100
11:15 AM	170/98
11:30 AM	164/94

Day 3—11:00 AM	
Lying	178/100
Sitting	166/90
Standing	150/90

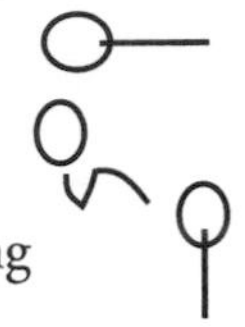

Interactive Activity: Record the blood pressure readings on the flow sheet using the symbol "**V**" to identify the systolic reading and the symbol "**Λ**" for the diastolic reading. Connect both symbols with a straight line. Identify the orthostatic blood pressure readings with the appropriate symbols. Compare your flow sheet with a partner.

Blood Pressure Flow Sheet

Date	Day 1			Day 2			Day 3		
Time	11:00	11:15	11:30	11:00	11:15	11:30	11:00		
240									
230									
220									
210									
200									
190									
180									
170									
160									
150									
140									
130									
120									
110									
100									
90									
80									
70									

APPLYING CRITICAL THINKING SKILLS TO TEST QUESTIONS

INSTRUCTIONS: Circle the one best answer for each test question. Write your rationale for selecting the answer. To enhance your learning and test-taking skills, discuss your answer and rationale with a partner. The answer and the rationale can be found on the back of this page.

1. The nurse is preparing to take the blood pressure of an adult patient for the first time. After placing the cuff on the patient's upper arm, it is most important for the nurse to:
   a. wait 1 minute before taking the blood pressure.
   b. place the stethoscope at the antecubital space.
   c. inflate the cuff to 150 mm Hg.
   d. palpate the systolic pressure.

   Rationale for your selection: ______________________________

2. The nurse uses a Doppler device to obtain the blood pressure measurement. In documenting the findings, the nurse will record the:
   a. systolic measurement.
   b. systolic and diastolic measurements.
   c. diastolic measurement.
   d. auscultatory gap.

   Rationale for your selection: ______________________________

3. In which of the following clients would the nurse expect a decreased blood pressure? A client:
   a. who is very anxious about being in the hospital.
   b. scheduled for major surgery.
   c. with a severe head injury.
   d. who hemorrhaged after surgery.

   Rationale for your selection: ______________________________

ANSWER KEY FOR APPLYING CRITICAL THINKING SKILLS TO TEST QUESTIONS

HELPFUL HINTS: Read all test questions carefully. Identify key words in the question that will guide you in answering the question. In these test questions the key words to consider are "**first time,**" "**initial action,**" and "**most appropriate.**" Compare your rationale with the one in the test question.

1. The nurse is preparing to take the blood pressure of an adult patient for the first time. After placing the cuff on the patient's upper arm, it is most important for the nurse to:
   a. wait 1 minute before taking the blood pressure.
   b. place the stethoscope at the antecubital space.
   c. inflate the cuff to 150 mm Hg.
   (d.) palpate the systolic pressure.

   Rationale: The answer is (d). Palpating for the systolic pressure provides the nurse with information for inflating the cuff to ensure an accurate systolic reading. Although option (b) is an action that the nurse would do, it is not the initial action. Options (a) and (c) are not appropriate for this situation.

2. The nurse uses a Doppler device to obtain the blood pressure measurement. In documenting the findings, the nurse will record the:
   (a.) systolic measurement.
   b. systolic and diastolic measurements.
   c. diastolic measurement.
   d. auscultatory gap.

   Rationale: The answer is (a). Doppler devices amplify sounds. In finding the blood pressure only the systolic measurement can be obtained with the use of a Doppler device. Options (b), (c), and (d) are not possible options when using a Doppler device.

3. In which of the following clients would the nurse expect a decreased blood pressure? A client:
   a. who is very anxious about being in the hospital.
   b. scheduled for major surgery.
   c. with a severe head injury.
   (d.) who hemorrhaged after surgery.

   Rationale: The answer is (d). Conditions that decrease the blood volume also decrease the cardiac output, which contributes to a decrease in blood pressure. Options (a), (b), and (c) are conditions that cause vasoconstriction, which increases the blood pressure.

ONE

BODY MECHANICS

List the **factors** that affect a patient's ability to move and maintain body alignment:

1. ____________________
2. ____________________
____
____
3. ____________________
4. ____________________
5. ____________________
6. ____________________

Use the diagram to identify the **four basic principles** of body mechanics:

1. ____________________
2. ____________________
3. ____________________
4. ____________________

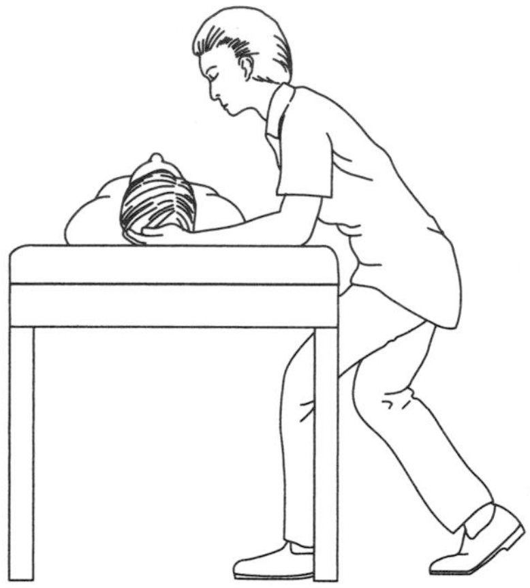

Case Study: The client has suffered a cerebral vascular accident (CVA) and as a result has left-sided hemiplegia. The physician orders the client to be out of bed (OOB) twice a day and to be turned every 2 hours while in bed. The RN asks the staff to do passive range of motion (ROM) exercises to the client's left side and to use supportive devices to ensure proper body alignment. The client is to be encouraged to do active ROM on the right side extremities.

Pertinent Terminology	Definition
Range of motion	
Active ROM	
Passive ROM	
CVA	
Hemiplegia	
Alignment	
Hand roll	
Trochanter roll	
Foot board	
Plantar flexion	
Flaccid	

From the case study, (1) **identify** the **major body areas** that would require special nursing care, (2) **select** the most appropriate **supportive device** from the list that will assist in maintaining proper body alignment for the client, and (3) **state** the **complication** the nursing care will help to prevent.

Hand roll	Trochanter roll	Pillow	Trapeze bar	Footboard

Major Body Area	Supportive Device	This helps to prevent
______________	______________	______________________
______________	______________	______________________
______________	______________	______________________
______________	______________	______________________
______________	______________	______________________

Select the activities of daily living (ADLs) below that the client can perform **independently** throughout the day that encourage **active ROM** to the **right side** of the body:

- ☐ Brushing teeth
- ☐ Transferring OOB
- ☐ Flexing/extending ankle
- ☐ Combing hair
- ☐ Ambulating
- ☐ Standing
- ☐ Washing face
- ☐ Feeding

Interactive Activity: With a partner, beginning with number 1, **number the following interventions** in the order necessary to assist the client to transfer from the bed to a wheelchair:

_____ Place wheelchair at a 45-degree angle to the bed.

_____ Lock the wheelchair brakes.

_____ Assist the client to a sitting position at the side of the bed.

_____ Provide instructions to the client.

_____ Cross left lower extremity over right lower extremity.

_____ Have the client pivot toward the wheelchair.

_____ Lower the client into the wheelchair.

_____ Stand the client; support left lower extremity.

_____ Have the client support left upper extremity with right upper extremity.

HYGIENE

The **purpose of providing a bath** is to:

1. ______________________
2. ______________________
3. ______________________
4. ______________________
5. ______________________

Identify the various types of baths:

1. ______________________
2. ______________________
3. ______________________
4. ______________________

Place a "✓" mark on the information that best describes the following.

Early morning care includes:

- ☐ Starting the bath early in the morning.
- ☐ Providing/assisting with oral hygiene.
- ☐ Washing face and hands.
- ☐ Offering bedpan, urinal, or assisting to the bathroom.

Hour of sleep (HS) care includes:

- ☐ Providing a back rub for the client.
- ☐ Straightening the bed linens.
- ☐ Providing/assisting with oral hygiene.
- ☐ Taking the vital signs.

Case Study: An 88-year-old female client has been in the hospital for 2 days with an irregular heartbeat. She is confused and just lies in bed. The RN informs you that the client has urinary and bowel incontinence and is wearing an adult incontinence pad. Her skin is very fragile, she has several ecchymotic areas on the lower extremities, she is wearing antiembolic stockings, and the pneumatic compression stockings are off. Her toenails are long, yellowish, and thick. She has dried feces under her fingernails.

Pertinent Terminology	Definition
Antiembolic stockings	
Pneumatic compression stockings	
Stomatitis	
Canthus	
Ecchymosis	
Perineum	
Labia majora	
Labia minora	
Prepuce	

Use the case study to identify the **most appropriate** nursing interventions for taking care of the client's hands and feet. **Circle** the nursing interventions below that you would implement:

Nursing Interventions:

Hands

1. Do nothing until the RN informs you.
2. Soak the hands for 10 minutes in lukewarm water.
3. Give the bath as usual, but do not soak the hands.
4. Use an orange stick or cotton swab to remove the feces.
5. Cut the fingernails carefully to prevent further collection under the nail beds.

Feet

1. Remove the antiembolic stockings during the bath.
2. Soak the feet for 10 minutes in lukewarm water.
3. Give a partial bath; apply lotion.
4. Dry well between the toes.
5. Cut the toenails carefully straight across.

Describe the proper method for performing perineal care on a:

Female: ____

____

Male: ____

____

Interactive Activity: With a partner, identify the type of bath **most appropriate** for the following case scenarios:

Case Scenarios	Type of Bath		
A 39-year-old woman who had abdominal surgery and will be discharged this morning	**Complete**	**Partial**	**Shower** (MD order/policy)
A 56-year-old patient admitted with lung problems who gets very short of breath with mild exertion	**Complete**	**Partial**	**Shower**
A 23-year-old woman who is alert but had a grand mal seizure 2 days ago	**Complete**	**Partial**	**Shower**
A 46-year-old patient who had a motor vehicle accident yesterday, had a mild concussion but no fractures	**Complete**	**Partial**	**Shower**

INFECTION CONTROL/TRANSMISSION OF ORGANISMS

Provide examples of the following elements found in the **chain of infection**:

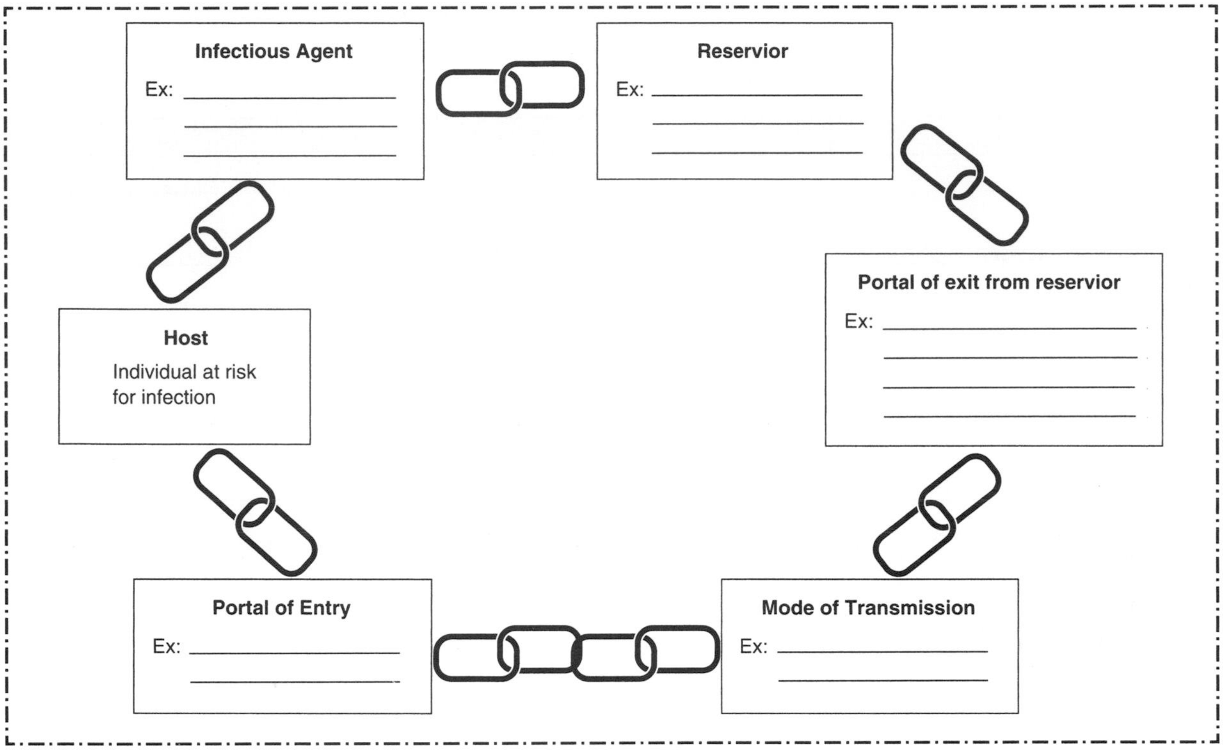

Case Study: A young woman has recently begun nursing school. During her second week in the clinical setting, she takes care of a 79-year-old client who was admitted with dehydration. The client has a recent history of shingles and is in the convalescent stage of illness. The client's skin is very dry, his oral temperature is 100.4° F. His urine is dark amber and his WBC is 13,000/mm^3.

Pertinent Terminology	Definition
Shingles	
Dehydration	
Incubation stage	
Prodromal stage	
Illness stage	
Convalescent stage	
Asepsis	
Nosocomial	
Iatrogenic	

From the case study, identify the **factors** that make the client susceptible for getting an infection.

______________________ ______________________

______________________ ______________________

Explain **why** each of the **factors** identified makes the client susceptible to getting an infection.

1. ______________________
2. ______________________
3. ______________________
4. ______________________

Define **medical asepsis:** ______________________

____

Define **surgical asepsis:** ______________________

____

In caring for the client, the nurse will use ______________ asepsis.

Interactive Activity: With a partner, fill in the **diagrams** with the proper **elements in the chain of infection** as it applies to each situation:

1. A family member who has a cold stops in to visit Mr. Wu.

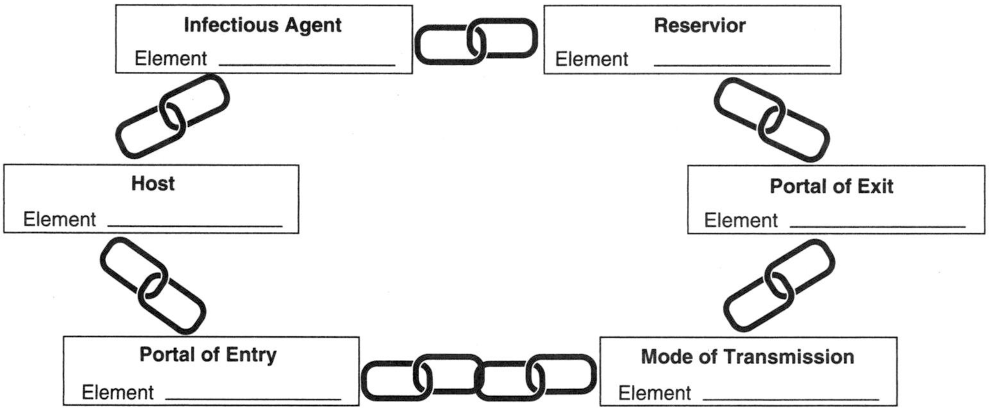

2. A nursing assistant goes from patient to patient without changing gloves.

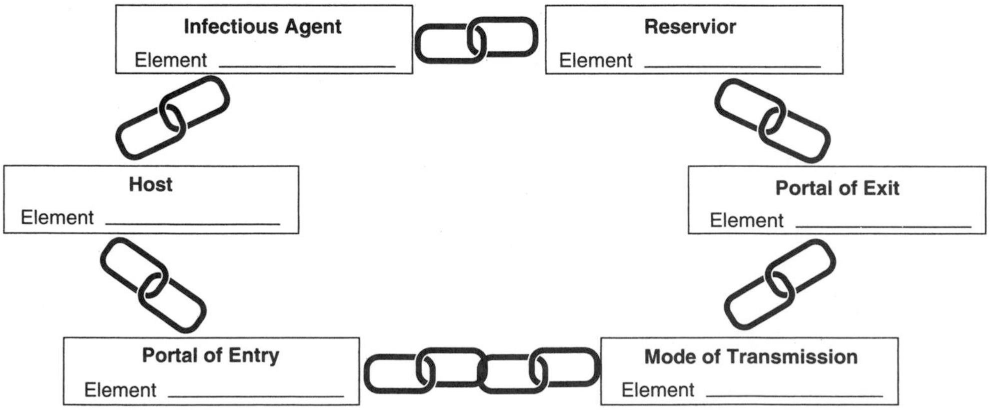

APPLYING CRITICAL THINKING SKILLS TO TEST QUESTIONS

INSTRUCTIONS: Circle the one best answer for each test question. Write your rationale for selecting the answer. To enhance your learning and test-taking skills, discuss your answer and rationale with a partner. The answer and the rationale can be found on the back of this page.

1. The nurse is taking care of a client who has a respiratory infection with a productive cough. The most effective infection control method is for the nurse to:
   a. monitor the temperature.
   b. push oral fluids every shift.
   c. have the client use a tissue when coughing.
   d. auscultate the lung sounds every 4 hours.

   Rationale for your selection: ______________________________

2. The client has been diagnosed with gastrointestinal bacteria obtained from drinking contaminated water. In the chain of infection, the water is the:
   a. portal of entry.
   b. reservoir.
   c. portal of exit.
   d. infectious agent.

   Rationale for your selection: ______________________________

3. The client's abdominal dressing is described as having a moderate amount of serosanguineous drainage and a very foul odor. In planning the dressing change, it is most important for the nurse to:
   a. apply extra dressings to the wound.
   b. use sterile gloves to change the dressing.
   c. wash her hands before and after the dressing change.
   d. change the abdominal dressing more often.

   Rationale for your selection: ______________________________

ANSWER KEY FOR APPLYING CRITICAL THINKING SKILLS TO TEST QUESTIONS

HELPFUL HINTS: Read all test questions carefully. Identify **key words** in the question that will guide you in answering the question. In these test questions the key words to consider are "**most effective,**" and "**most important.**" Compare your rationale with the one in the test question.

1. The nurse is taking care of a client who has a respiratory infection with a productive cough. The most effective infection control method is for the nurse to:
   a. monitor the temperature.
   b. push oral fluids every shift.
   (c.) have the client use a tissue when coughing.
   d. auscultate the lung sounds every 4 hours.

   Rationale: The answer is (c). Having the client use a tissue helps to stop the spread of infectious airborne pathogens. Options (a), (b), and (d) are good nursing interventions but are not effective in controlling infection.

2. The client has been diagnosed with gastrointestinal bacteria obtained from drinking contaminated water. In the chain of infection, the water is the:
   a. portal of entry.
   (b.) reservoir.
   c. portal of exit.
   d. infectious agent.

   Rationale: The answer is (b). The water is the reservoir that provided the environment for the infectious agent to reproduce. Options (a), (c), and (d) are part of the chain of infection, but the water is the reservoir.

3. The client's abdominal dressing is described as having a moderate amount of serosanguineous drainage and a very foul odor. In planning the dressing change, it is most important for the nurse to:
   a. apply extra dressings to the wound.
   b. use sterile gloves to change the dressing.
   (c.) wash her hands before and after the dressing change.
   d. change the abdominal dressing more often.

   Rationale: The answer is (c). Hand washing is the single most effective method in preventing the spread of pathogens. Option (a) can be done, but it is not the most important option; options (b) and (d) are ordered by the practitioner.

SKIN INTEGRITY

List the **factors** that increase the **risk** for development of a pressure ulcer:

1. ______________________
2. ______________________
3. ______________________
4. ______________________
5. ______________________
6. ______________________
7. ______________________
8. ______________________
9. ______________________
10. ______________________
11. ______________________

Use the diagram to **circle** the areas of the body where **pressure ulcers** are likely to develop on a bedridden patient:

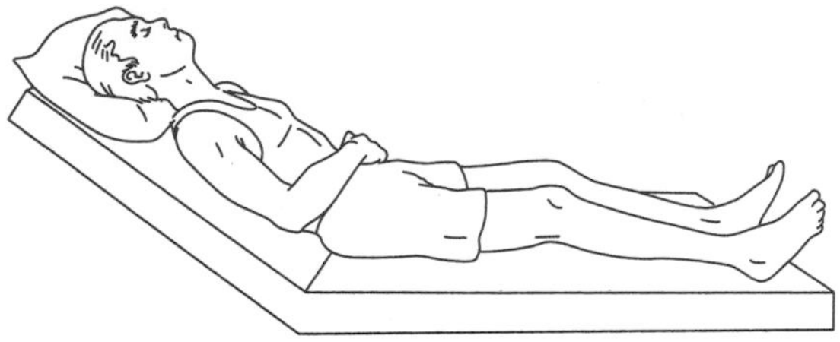

Case Study: An 88-year-old female client has been admitted to the hospital with a fractured left elbow. She is malnourished and weighs only 90 pounds. She is currently confused and the physician has ordered a vest restraint to prevent her from falling out of bed. The family reports that the client eats less than 50% of her meals and has difficulty walking. The client is anorexic and her skin is soft and thin. She is incontinent of urine.

Pertinent Terminology	Definition
Pressure ulcer	
Necrosis	
Ischemia	
Reactive hyperemia	
Blanching	
Slough	
Eschar	
Tunneling	
Debridement	
Excoriation	

BRADEN SCALE FOR PREDICTING PRESSURE SORE RISK

Visit *http://evolve.elsevier.com/castillo/thinking* for an interactive activity using the Braden Scale where you will **select the number** that best applies to the client's risk for development of pressure ulcers (the **lower the number**, the greater is the risk for the development of pressure ulcers).

- After 2 days of taking care of the client, the nurse made the following documentation on the client's chart: "Reddened, open, dry circular area on sacrum, approximately 2.5 cm × 2.5 cm. Dr. Stanley notified."
- Use the documentation to check off (✓) the "**stage**" of the client's pressure ulcer from the **Pressure Ulcer Stages** below:

Suspected Deep Tissue Injury

☐ Purple or maroon discolored area; intact skin or blood-filled blister

Stage I

☐ Nonblanchable redness of a localized area; intact skin.

Stage II

☐ Partial-thickness dermal loss. Pink wound bed without slough. May present as an intact or open serum-filled blister.

Stage III

☐ Full-thickness tissue loss; subcutaneous tissue may be visible, but bone, tendon, or muscle are not exposed. Slough, tunneling, and undermining may be present.

Stage IV

☐ Full-thickness tissue loss with exposed bone, tendon, or muscle. Slough and eschar may be present on some parts of the wound bed. Tunneling and undermining may also be present.

Unstageable

☐ Full-thickness tissue loss in which the base of the ulcer is covered by slough or eschar.

Interactive Activity: With a partner, **write in** the "**stage**" of the pressure ulcer for each of the following case studies using the **Pressure Ulcer Stages**:

Case Study	Pressure Ulcer Stage
A male client was brought to the hospital. He has an open wound on his left heel that is 2 inches wide and ½ inch deep. It has a foul odor and the heel bone is exposed.	____________
The nurse measures an irregular open wound on the right hip. The subcutaneous tissue is visible.	____________

For a continuation of this case study, go to *http://evolve.elsevier.com/castillo/thinking.*

APPLYING CRITICAL THINKING SKILLS TO TEST QUESTIONS

INSTRUCTIONS: Circle the one best answer for each test question. Write your rationale for selecting the answer. To enhance your learning and test-taking skills, discuss your answer and rationale with a partner. The answer and the rationale can be found on the back of this page.

1. The nurse is taking care of a client who has a stage I pressure ulcer on the sacrum. In delegating the care of the client, it is most important for the nurse to:
   a. instruct the nursing assistant to turn the client every 2 hours.
   b. ask the nursing assistant to massage the client's sacrum.
   c. review how to assess the client's sacrum with the nursing assistant.
   d. inform the nursing assistant of the client's pressure ulcer.

   Rationale for your selection: ______________________________

2. While reading the chart of a client, the nurse notes that the physician has identified eschar on the left heel. Which of the following assessments is most significant of this finding?
   a. A black scabbed-like area on the left heel
   b. A bruised area on the left heel
   c. A stage III pressure ulcer on the left heel
   d. A stage IV pressure ulcer on the left heel

   Rationale for your selection: ______________________________

3. On turning a client to the lateral position, the nurse notes a reddened area on the right hip. Further assessment reveals intact skin with blanching at the site. Which of the following is the most appropriate nursing intervention?
   a. Notify the physician.
   b. Document the findings.
   c. Apply a dry sterile dressing.
   d. Document the presence of a stage I pressure ulcer.

   Rationale for your selection: ______________________________

ANSWER KEY FOR APPLYING CRITICAL THINKING SKILLS TO TEST QUESTIONS

HELPFUL HINTS: Read all test questions carefully. Identify key words in the question that will guide you in answering the question. In these test questions the **key words** to consider are **"most important," "most significant,"** and **"most appropriate."** Compare your rationale with the one in the test question.

1. The nurse is taking care of a client who has a stage I pressure ulcer on the sacrum. In delegating the care of the client, it is most important for the nurse to:
   (a.) instruct the nursing assistant to turn the client every 2 hours.
   b. ask the nursing assistant to massage the client's sacrum.
   c. review how to assess the client's sacrum with the nursing assistant.
   d. inform the nursing assistant of the client's pressure ulcer.

   Rationale: The answer is (a). Instructing the nursing assistant to carry out an intervention that would assist in preventing further skin breakdown is most important. Option (b) could cause more tissue damage; option (c) is not appropriate for a nursing assistant to assess, and option (d) is not client centered nor provides a specific intervention to assist the client.

2. While reading the chart of a client, the nurse notes that the physician has identified eschar on the left heel. Which of the following assessments is most significant of this finding?
   (a.) A black scabbed-like area on the left heel
   b. A bruised area on the left heel
   c. A stage III pressure ulcer on the left heel
   d. A stage IV pressure ulcer on the left heel

   Rationale: The answer is (a), which describes the appearance of eschar. Eschar must be debrided to "stage" the pressure ulcer. Options (b), (c), and (d) do not describe the finding.

3. On turning a client to the lateral position, the nurse notes a reddened area on the right hip. Further assessment reveals intact skin with blanching at the site. Which of the following is the most appropriate nursing intervention?
   a. Notify the physician.
   (b.) Document the findings.
   c. Apply a dry sterile dressing.
   d. Document the presence of a stage I pressure ulcer.

   Rationale: The answer is (b). A reddened area with intact skin and blanching indicates circulation to the site. Options (a) and (c) are not necessary at this time. For option (d), the findings do not support the definition of a stage I pressure ulcer.

COMMUNICATION

List essential **therapeutic communication techniques** used in a helping relationship:

- ____________________ • ____________________
- ____________________ • ____________________
- ____________________ • ____________________
- ____________________ • ____________________
- ____________________ • ____________________

Identify **nontherapeutic responses** that block the development of therapeutic communication:

- ______________________________
- ______________________________
- ______________________________
- ______________________________
- ______________________________
- ______________________________

Use the diagrams to identify the **factors** that influence communication:

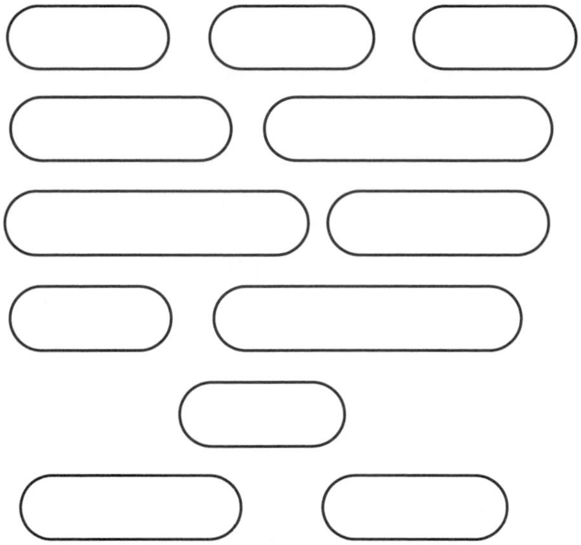

Case Study: Casey, a student nurse, is in the clinical facility for the first time. She is assigned to a 70-year-old female client who was admitted with a fracture of the right hip. The client had her own business for 30 years but is now retired. She remains active in her community. The staff tells the student nurse that the client is a very cranky woman. As soon as Casey walks into the room she hears: "Well, it is about time! If I had to wait any longer I probably would starve to death." Casey responds softly, "I just came on duty."

Pertinent Terminology	Definition
Therapeutic relationship	
Orientation phase	
Testing	
Working phase	
Termination phase	
Paraphrasing	
Open-ended question	

Use the case study to identify **three factors** that would initially affect the development of a therapeutic relationship with the client:

________________ ________________ ________________

Casey's response to the client is an example of ________________________.

Casey may have addressed the client's statements by saying: ________________________

Identify the **therapeutic communication technique** used by Casey in the statement and provide a **rationale** as to why this statement is more appropriate:

Therapeutic Technique	**Rationale**
________________	________________________

Interactive Activity: With a partner, use the following scenarios to select the appropriate communication technique or response being used:

Paraphrasing	False reassurance	Summarizing
Open-ended question	Clarification	Opinion

1. **Nurse:** "Good morning Mr. S, I heard you had a lot of pain last night. Could you describe the type of pain you had?"

   ____

2. **Family Member:** "The doctor just told me that my husband suffered a severe heart attack!"

   Nurse: "I'm sorry, but don't worry, I'm sure everything will be fine."

   ____

3. **Client:** "I'm just so sick all the time. I just can't do anything by myself anymore. I feel so helpless!"

   Nurse: "It is hard for you to be so dependent and not feel like you are in control. You sound pretty tired of it all."

   ____

4. **Client:** "Nurse, I need to know more information on the pill you gave me this morning."

   Nurse: "Mr. G, I gave you several pills this morning. Which one would you like to know more about?"

   ____

APPLYING CRITICAL THINKING SKILLS TO TEST QUESTIONS

INSTRUCTIONS: Circle the one best answer for each test question. Write your rationale for selecting the answer. To enhance your learning and test-taking skills, discuss your answer and rationale with a partner. The answer and the rationale can be found on the back of this page.

1. The following conversation takes place at the client's bedside:
   Nurse: "Good morning Mr. J., I am your nurse for today. Did you sleep well?"
   Client: "I am not sure."
   Nurse: "You are not sure?"
   Which of the following statements is most accurate of this conversation? The nurse:
   a. should ask a question to validate the client's confusion.
   b. used an appropriate follow-up communication technique.
   c. should look at the chart to see how the client slept.
   d. was inappropriate in asking the second question.

   Rationale for your selection: ______________________________
   ____
   ____
   ____
   ____

2. The nurse walks into a client's room and sees the postsurgical client holding his abdomen and grimacing. The nurse states, "You look like you are in pain." The nurse's statement is:
   a. appropriate because it states what the nurse is observing.
   b. appropriate because pain is expected after surgery.
   c. inappropriate because the nurse made a conclusion before validating.
   d. inappropriate because the nurse should wait for the client to speak first.

   Rationale for your selection: ______________________________
   ____
   ____
   ____
   ____

3. The following conversation takes place at the client's bedside:
   Nurse: "Mr. T, I will be teaching you how to change your surgical dressing."
   Client: "I would prefer that you wait until my wife gets here. She takes care of everything."
   Nurse: "You shouldn't depend on your wife. I'll show you first and then you can teach your wife."
   The nurse's last statement is:
   a. displaying a value judgment.
   b. appropriate because it encourages self-care.
   c. having the client reinforce what will be taught.
   d. inappropriate because that nurse should have called the wife first.

   Rationale for your selection: ______________________________
   ____
   ____
   ____
   ____

ANSWER KEY FOR APPLYING CRITICAL THINKING SKILLS TO TEST QUESTIONS

HELPFUL HINTS: Read all test questions carefully. Identify key words in the question that will guide you in answering the question. In these test questions the **key words** to consider are **"most accurate,"** and **"most important."** Compare your rationale with the one in the test question.

1. The following conversation takes place at the client's bedside:
   Nurse: "Good morning Mr. J., I am your nurse for today. Did you sleep well?"
   Client: "I am not sure."
   Nurse: "You are not sure?"
   Which of the following statements is most accurate of this conversation? The nurse:
   a. should ask a question to validate the client's confusion.
   (b.) used an appropriate follow-up communication technique.
   c. should look at the chart to see how the client slept.
   d. was inappropriate in asking the second question.

   Rationale: The answer is (b). The nurse used a reflective (paraphrase) technique to solicit more information from the client. Options (a), (c), and (d) do not solicit more information.

2. The nurse walks into a client's room and sees the postsurgical client holding his abdomen and grimacing. The nurse states, "You look like you are in pain." The nurse's statement is:
   (a.) appropriate because it states what the nurse is observing.
   b. appropriate because pain is expected after surgery.
   c. inappropriate because the nurse made a conclusion before validating.
   d. inappropriate because the nurse should wait for the client to speak first.

   Rationale: The answer is (a). The nurse is stating the objective observations. This allows the client to clarify or validate the observation. Options (b), (c), and (d) are not appropriate therapeutic communication techniques that facilitate client communication.

3. The following conversation takes place at the client's bedside:
   Nurse: "Mr. T, I will be teaching you how to change your surgical dressing."
   Client: "I would prefer that you wait until my wife gets here. She takes care of everything."
   Nurse: "You shouldn't depend on your wife. I'll show you first and then you can teach your wife."
   The nurse's last statement is:
   (a.) displaying a value judgment.
   b. appropriate because it encourages self-care.
   c. having the client reinforce what will be taught.
   d. inappropriate because that nurse should have called the wife first.

   Rationale: The answer is (a). The nurse's comment reflects how the nurse feels about the client's decision. This can cause a block to communication. Options (b), (c), and (d) do not take into consideration the importance of the client's personal needs and social structure.

REPORTING PATIENT STATUS

List the most common methods nurses use to **report patient status** during the shift and from shift to shift:

1. ______________________
2. ______________________
3. ______________________
4. ______________________

Place an "X" in the box(es) that best describe(s) the information that should be included in a **change-of-shift report**. The change-of-shift report should:

- ☐ Provide basic information such as room number, date of admission, and medical diagnosis.
- ☐ Provide specific information regarding the client's needs.
- ☐ Provide information on significant changes in the client's condition.
- ☐ Provide information on follow-up client care.
- ☐ Provide information on clients transferred or discharged from the unit (varies in some hospitals).

Case Study: 0700 (RN, change of shift morning report on the following two patients)

"Mr. J in room 461 is a 76-year-old man. He was admitted last night with sepsis. He has an IV of D5W infusing at 75 mL/hr. He is NPO. His output for the shift is 150 mL total. The 0600 temperature is 100.6° F and his blood pressure is 146/94. I am concerned about his temperature and output, so I think it is important to monitor his output and temperature every 4 hours."

"Mr. H in room 462 has been here for 3 days with pneumonia. His temperature at 0600 was 102.4° F and I gave him two Tylenol tablets. His pulse oximetry was 94% on room air. He has an IV infusing at 100 mL/hr and there are 300 mL left. He has a productive cough and is bringing up thick whitish phlegm. I sent the sputum specimen to the laboratory. He has taken in only 50 mL of oral fluid and his output was 275 mL for the shift. I recommend that his temperature be monitored every 2 hours throughout the shift and his intake be discussed with his doctor today."

Pertinent Terminology	Definition
Nursing Rand/Kardex	
Worksheet	
Reporting	
SBAR	

Use the **case study** to fill in the worksheet with the pertinent information obtained in morning report on the clients:

Worksheet

Pt. Name: ____________ Age: ______ VS: ______________ ______________ Amb. _____ Bed rest _____ Bath (self) ___ (Bed) _____	Rm: _____ I = _____ O = _____ Diet: _____	Dx: __________ Admit date _______ IV: __________ __________ __________	Follow-up Notes: __________ __________ __________ __________ __________ __________
Pt. Name: ____________ Age: ______ VS: ______________ Pulse ox: __________ Amb. _____ Bed rest _____ Bath (self) ___ (Bed) _____	Rm: _____ I = _____ O = _____ Diet: _____	Dx: __________ Admit date _______ IV: __________ __________ __________	Follow-up Notes: __________ __________ __________ __________ __________ __________ __________

Additional information to **complete the worksheet is found** in the ____________________.

Interactive Activity: With a partner, answer the questions regarding (1) the **change-of-shift report** for the following case study and (2) **fill in the worksheet** and discuss the **follow-up notes:**

1500 (**change-of-shift** report)
"Mr. W, 92 years old, in room 357 was admitted yesterday with anemia. His hemoglobin this morning is 7.2 mg/dL and his hematocrit is 26%. He is hard of hearing and weighs 127 pounds. His Foley catheter drained only 100 mL all shift. He has an IV of normal saline solution infusing at 75 mL/hr. He will receive 2 units of blood this evening. The lab will call when the blood is ready. The family and client will make a decision soon regarding his code status. He is very weak and needs a lot of assistance."

- **Identify the basic information** given in the report: ______________________________
____

- **Identify the significant information** given in the report: ______________________________
____
____

Worksheet

Pt. Name: ____________ Age: ______ VS: ______________ ______________ Amb. _____ Bed rest _____ Bath (self) ___ (Bed) _____	Rm: _____ I = _____ O = _____ Diet: _____	Dx: __________ Admit date _______ IV: __________ __________ __________	Follow-up Notes: __________ __________ __________ __________ __________ __________

For a continuation of this case study, go to *http://evolve.elsevier.com/castillo/thinking*.

INTRODUCTION TO THE ASSESSMENT PROCESS

List the **methods** available to the nurse for the **collection of patient data:**

1. ____________________
2. ____________________
3. ____________________
4. ____________________

List the **parts of the patient's chart** that assist the nurse in the **collection of patient data:**

1. ____________________
2. ____________________
3. ____________________
4. ____________________
5. ____________________
6. ____________________

Draw a line to connect the **Objective Data.**

Subjective

"I have a headache."

Gold-colored chain

States nauseated

Resp. 22 regular

WBC is 5,000/mm^3

Objective

Case Study: Mrs. C has been admitted to the hospital for the birth of her baby. Her husband is by her side. You observe that she is very pleasant but cries out with each contraction. She tells you, "I feel a lot of pressure in my back." Her chart indicates that she is 26 years old and that she has a 6-year-old son.

Pertinent Terminology	Definition
Assessment	
Subjective data	
Objective data	
Clustering data	
Validation of data	
Primary source	
Secondary source	

Use the case study to identify the following information:

List the **objective data:**	**Source (Primary/Secondary)**
1. ______________________________	
2. ______________________________	____________
3. ______________________________	____________
4. ______________________________	____________

List the **subjective data:**

1. ______________________________ ____________

Interactive Activity: With a partner, **use the box to identify subjective and objective data** from the case studies:

Mrs. T has been admitted with depression. She answers questions softly with a "yes" or "no" response. She wants her door closed and her room dark. She refuses visitors and eats only 10% of her meals. You notice that she cries regularly and sleeps a lot. She bites her nails frequently.

Objective Data

____
____
____
____
____
____
____

Subjective Data

____
____

Mr. P had surgery 1 day ago. He tells you that he has been very independent all his life and hates being sick. He has refused his pain medication all morning. You notice that he refuses to get out of bed, he moans quietly every now and then, he is sweaty, and his hands are clenched tightly. His surgical dressing is clean and he says everything is fine when you ask him a question.

Objective Data

____
____
____
____
____
____
____

Subjective Data

____
____

Mr. K informs the nursing assistant that he is nauseated. He has refused his lunch. You go in to check him and you notice 100 mL of clear yellow emesis. He tells you that he vomited. His wife is at his bedside.

Objective Data

____
____
____
____
____
____
____

Subjective Data

____
____

BASIC PHYSICAL ASSESSMENT

List the **four methods of examination** used in the performance of a physical assessment:

1. ______________________
2. ______________________
3. ______________________
4. ______________________

Write in the most appropriate **method of examination**(s) for each of the following:

- Oral mucous membranes ______________________
- Peripheral pulses ______________________
- Arterial blood pressure ______________________
- Lung sounds ______________________
- Lower extremity edema ______________________
- Apical pulse ______________________
- Distended abdomen ______________________

Case Study: Carrie is a nursing student assigned to Ms. W. Ms. W, 18 years old, came to the emergency department with complaints of right lower abdominal pains. She was admitted and had an appendectomy the day of admission. She is 2 days postop and will be going home this afternoon. Carrie performs a **body systems assessment** and documents the following notes:

Neuro: Alert and oriented × 3. **Cardiovascular:** Radial pulse regular and bounding. **Skin:** Warm and dry, pallor present, turgor elastic. **Respirations:** Regular, clear. **Gastrointestinal:** Bowel sounds present in all four quadrants. RLQ abdominal dressing clean, complains of tenderness with light palpation. **Genitourinary:** States voiding without difficulty. **Musculoskeletal:** Ambulates with a steady gait. **Psychosocial:** Cheerful.

Pertinent Terminology	Definition
Inspection	
Palpation	
Percussion	
Auscultation	
Chief complaint	
Review of systems	

Use the documentation notes from the case study to **identify the method of examination** used by Carrie in performing the body systems assessment:

Documentation	Method(s) of Examination
• **Neuro:** Alert and oriented × 3	______________________
• **Cardiovascular:** Radial pulse regular and bounding	______________________
• **Skin:** Warm and dry, pallor, turgor elastic	______________________
• **Respirations:** Regular, clear	______________________
• **Gastrointestinal:** Bowel sounds present in all four quadrants. Right lower quadrant abdominal dressing clean, complains of tenderness with light palpation	______________________
• **Genitourinary:** States voiding without difficulty	______________________
• **Musculoskeletal:** Ambulates with a steady gait	______________________
• **Psychosocial:** Cheerful	______________________

Interactive Activity: With a partner, use the following documentation notes to (1) **identify** the **body system** being assessed and (2) **the method of examination** used:

Documentation Notes	Body System/Method(s) of Examination
States it is 1945, does not know where he is; knows first name; hand grips unequal right < left	______________________ ______________________
Voided 50 mL of amber fluid; abdomen distended	______________________ ______________________
Warm, moist; pallor with erythema on sacral area; edema 1+ on bilateral lower extremities	______________________ ______________________
Absent bowel sounds in lower and upper right quadrants, hyperactive on upper and lower left quadrant; having small amounts of liquid dark brown stools	______________________ ______________________
Wheezes audible on inspiration, coughing, expectorating thick yellowish phlegm	______________________ ______________________
Apical pulse 116, rapid, irregular; radial pulse 98, rapid, thready, irregular	______________________ ______________________
Passive range of motion to right hand. Unable to extend and flex fingers	______________________ ______________________
Left facial drooping; left arm and leg flaccid	______________________ ______________________

APPLYING CRITICAL THINKING SKILLS TO TEST QUESTIONS

INSTRUCTIONS: Circle the one best answer for each test question. Write your rationale for selecting the answer. To enhance your learning and test-taking skills, discuss your answer and rationale with a partner. The answer and the rationale can be found on the back of this page.

1. The nurse is preparing to assess the neurologic status of an adult client who had a hip fracture 5 days ago and was reported to have been confused the previous shift. Which statement will provide the nurse with the most appropriate information?
   a. "Can you tell me today's date."
   b. "Do you know that you are in the hospital?"
   c. "When did you have hip surgery?"
   d. "Tell me where you are right now."

   Rationale for your selection: ______________________________

2. The nurse is informed that a newly admitted client is complaining of itching and has a rash all over the body. The most appropriate nursing intervention initially is to:
   a. inform the physician of the objective and subjective complaints.
   b. inspect the client and describe the rash.
   c. ask the client to try not to scratch the areas.
   d. check the medication record for anti-itch medication.

   Rationale for your selection: ______________________________

3. The nurse is assigned to a client who was admitted for a blood clot in the right leg. Which of the following describes the appropriate assessment technique initially?
   a. Inspection of the right leg
   b. Light palpation of the right leg
   c. Inspection followed by deep palpation of edematous areas
   d. Light palpation followed by inspection of any reddened areas

   Rationale for your selection: ______________________________

ANSWER KEY FOR APPLYING CRITICAL THINKING SKILLS TO TEST QUESTIONS

HELPFUL HINTS: Read all test questions carefully. Identify key words in the question that will guide you in answering the question. In these test questions the **key words** to consider are "**most appropriate**" and "**initially.**" Compare your rationale with the one in the test question.

1. The nurse is preparing to assess the neurologic status of an adult client who had a hip fracture 5 days ago and was reported to have been confused the previous shift. Which statement will provide the nurse with the most appropriate information?
   a. "Can you tell me today's date."
   b. "Do you know that you are in the hospital?"
   c. "When did you have hip surgery?"
   (d.) "Tell me where you are right now."

   Rationale: The answer is (d). Eliciting orientation to place is part of assessing client orientation. Options (a) and (b) encourage a "yes" or "no" response, and option (c) may not give accurate data if the client does not remember the date.

2. The nurse is informed that a newly admitted client is complaining of itching and has a rash all over the body. The most appropriate nursing intervention initially is to:
   a. inform the physician of the objective and subjective complaints.
   (b.) inspect the client and describe the rash.
   c. ask the client to try not to scratch the areas.
   d. check the medication record for anti-itch medication.

   Rationale: The answer is (b). It is most appropriate for the nurse to initially gather data by using the assessment skill of inspection and then to further describe the observations. Options (a), (c), and (d) are follow-up nursing interventions.

3. The nurse is assigned to a client who was admitted for a blood clot in the right leg. Which of the following describes the appropriate assessment technique initially?
   (a.) Inspection of the right leg
   b. Light palpation of the right leg
   c. Inspection followed by deep palpation of edematous areas
   d. Light palpation followed by inspection of any reddened areas

   Rationale: The answer is (a). Inspection is the initial step in the assessment process that provides information on color, size, shape, and movement of the extremity. Options (b) and (d) are not appropriate initially, and option (c) should not be done in this situation.

DOCUMENTATION

List the primary documentation (charting) formats used in the clinical settings:

1. ______________________________
2. ______________________________
3. ______________________________
4. ______________________________
5. ______________________________
6. ______________________________

Circle the statements that are **true**.

The chart is a communication tool.

The RN is legally responsible for the documentation made by student nurses.

Charting entries should be concise.

Flow sheets are not part of the client's chart.

Pertinent Terminology	Definition
APIE charting	
Charting by exception	
Clinical pathways	
Electronic charting	
Narrative charting	
Flow sheets	
Focus charting	
POMR charting	
SOAP charting	

Review the Clinical Pathway at *http://evolve.elsevier.com/castillo/thinking* and the Nurses' Notes below to correlate interventions and documentation.

Example #1

Nurses' Notes	
Time	
0800	Alert, oriented ×4. States pain level 5 using PCA. Lung sounds clear, unlabored using incentive spirometer Skin warm, dry. NG to suction draining light brown. BS absent ×4 quads. Abd dressing with 2 cm × 2 cm pinkish drainage. ———— M. Molly RN
0900	Foley discontinued as ordered. ———— M. Molly RN

Charting format: ________________

Example #2

ADL Documentation					
Time	0930				
Initials	MM				
Hygiene:					
Bath		Bed	Assisted	Self	Shower
Oral care		Self		Assisted	
Pericare		Self		Cath	
Diet					
Intake		Brkft	Lunch	Dinner	
%		0			
Fed		Self	Assisted	NPO	
Mobility					
Ambulation		Independent		Assisted	
		Chair		BR	

Charting format: ________________

Interactive Activity: With a partner, use the following **Nurses' Notes** to identify five documentation errors. List how these errors should be corrected.

Nurses' Notes	
Time	
0700	Sleeping. Resp.20 reg. unlabored. Skin warm ——————————— M. Molly RN
0730	Awake, pain level 0. Patient up to bathroom MAEW. c/o dizziness on returning to bed. Pale assisted back to bed. P 98, irregular. BP 90/60 no c/o pain. Side rails up ×4. —— M. Molly RN
0830	Refused breakfast, c/o mild indegestion. Will check to see what medications are ordered ——— M. Molly RN

Charting errors:

1. ______________________________

   Correct by: ______________________________

2. ______________________________

   Correct by: ______________________________

3. ______________________________

   Correct by: ______________________________

4. ______________________________

   Correct by: ______________________________

5. ______________________________

   Correct by: ______________________________

For a continuation of this case study, go to *http://evolve.elsevier.com/castillo/thinking*.

SELF-CONCEPT

List the **four components** of self-concept:

1. ______________________
2. ______________________
3. ______________________
4. ______________________

For each of the **self-concept** components, **identify two stressors** that affect and contribute to altering the component of:

➢ **Identity** (any two)

____

____

➢ **Body image** (any two)

____

____

____

➢ **Self-esteem** (any two)

____

____

____

➢ **Role performance** (any two)

____

____

Case Study: A female client was diagnosed with breast cancer 2 weeks ago and recently had a left mastectomy. She is 32 years old and is married with a 5-year-old daughter. She is very anxious after the surgery and wonders how her husband will react to her. She tells the nurse, "I am so young to have this done." She begins to cry and says that she loves being a mom but doesn't think she can have another child because she would not be able to nurse and care for the baby as she would like to. She is scheduled to begin chemotherapy treatments in 1 week.

Pertinent Terminology	Definition
Self-concept	
Identity	
Body image	
Self-esteem	
Role performance	

Reread the case study and cluster the **objective data** and **subjective data** that relate to the **self-concept** component that is marked with an "X":

- ☐ Identity
- ☒ **Body image**
- ☐ Self-esteem
- ☐ Role performance

➡ **Objective data:**

➡ **Subjective data:**

- ☐ Identity
- ☐ Body image
- ☐ Self-esteem
- ☒ **Role performance**

➡ **Objective data:**

➡ **Subjective data:**

Interactive Activity: With a partner, use the following case study to cluster the objective data and the subjective data related to the **self-concept** component that is marked with an "X":

Case Study

A male client suffered a heart attack 2 months ago and has lost his job. When he comes to the clinic, his facial expression is tense and he speaks in a hostile voice. During the last visit, he stated: "I can't just sit here, I am the breadwinner of my family." "I'm useless since I had the heart attack!"

- ☒ **Identity**
- ☐ Body image
- ☐ Self-esteem
- ☐ Role performance

➡ **Objective data:**

➡ **Subjective data:**

- ☐ Identity
- ☐ Body image
- ☒ **Self-esteem**
- ☐ Role performance

➡ **Objective data:**

➡ **Subjective data:**

CULTURAL ASPECTS OF NURSING

List the **six cultural phenomena** that influence nursing care:

1. ______________________
2. ______________________
3. ______________________
4. ______________________
5. ______________________
6. ______________________

List **two examples** for each of the following:

Communication
1. ______________________
2. ______________________

Social organizations
1. ______________________
2. ______________________

Environmental control
1. ______________________
2. ______________________

Biologic variations
1. ______________________
2. ______________________

Case Study: Wendy RN, the home health nurse, visits a 62-year-old Hispanic woman who has had diabetes mellitus for 20 years and currently has a sore on her left foot. The client has missed two of her doctor's appointments and has been soaking her foot in warm salt water every night. The client speaks English but does not like to call the clinic or question the nurse because she does want to bother anyone. She enjoys cooking and eating Mexican food. During the home visit Wendy noticed several religious artifacts and many pictures of the client's children and grandchildren on the wall.

Pertinent Terminology	Definition
Culture	
Culture shock	
Cultural sensitivity	
Ethnicity	
Acculturation	
Ethnocentrism	
Transcultural nursing	

Use the case study to **identify** the **cultural data** that relates to the **culture phenomena** listed below:

Culture Phenomena	Cultural Data
Communication	
Space	
Time	
Social organization	
Environmental control	
Biologic variation	

Interactive Activity: With a partner, use the following case studies to (1) **underline** the pertinent **cultural data** and (2) **identify** the **possible implications** for health care delivery:

Case Study	Health Care Delivery Implication(s)
A Filipino woman, is very quiet. She rarely complains, and the nurses comment on how she doesn't maintain eye contact when the nurse is speaking.	
A client of Chinese ancestry is 80 years old and requires constant care. She lives with one of her daughters, and all the adult family members are involved in caring for her at night.	
Mrs. W has had a miscarriage. She hemorrhaged and her blood count is very low. The physician has recommended a blood transfusion, but Mrs. W refuses because of her religious beliefs.	
An African-American woman comes to the outpatient clinic for blood pressure checks. She tells the nurse that her youngest daughter is about to be married. She is concerned because her other daughter has sickle cell anemia.	
A male client had major surgery yesterday. He does not want to get out of bed and has refused all his pain medication. The nurse knows that he is in pain but wants to respect his wishes.	

APPLYING CRITICAL THINKING SKILLS TO TEST QUESTIONS

INSTRUCTIONS: Circle the one best answer for each test question. Write your rationale for selecting the answer. To enhance your learning and test-taking skills, discuss your answer and rationale with a partner. The answer and the rationale can be found on the back of this page.

1. The nurse is asking an alert elderly Hispanic female client to sign a consent for a bronchoscopy procedure scheduled the next day. The client tells the nurse that she wants to wait until her family arrives later. Which nursing action is most appropriate?
   a. Ask the client to sign but inform her that she can change her mind.
   b. Ask the client if she has any questions you can answer.
   c. Tell the client to call you when her family arrives.
   d. Inform the physician.

   Rationale for your selection: ______________________________

2. The nurse is taking care of a client who is scheduled for surgery today. The client asks the nurse to read a passage from the Bible to help her prepare herself for surgery. It is most appropriate for the nurse to:
   a. read the Bible passage.
   b. ask if someone on staff is the same religion as the client.
   c. kindly tell the client that nurses cannot get involved in religious issues.
   d. inquire whether the client would prefer that a religious person be called.

   Rationale for your selection: ______________________________

3. The nurse is assigned to a client who believes that wearing a copper bracelet will relieve arthritic pain. In providing care for the client, it is most important for the nurse to:
   a. encourage the client to use anti-inflammatory medication.
   b. inform the client that copper bracelets have no proven medical value.
   c. address the pathophysiologic mechanisms associated with arthritis with the client.
   d. respect the beliefs associated with the copper bracelet by the client.

   Rationale for your selection: ______________________________

ANSWER KEY FOR APPLYING CRITICAL THINKING SKILLS TO TEST QUESTIONS

HELPFUL HINTS: Read all test questions carefully. Identify key words in the question that will guide you in answering the question. In these test questions the **key words** to consider are **"most appropriate"** and **"most important."** Compare your rationale with the one in the test question.

1. The nurse is asking an alert elderly Hispanic female client to sign a consent for a bronchoscopy procedure scheduled the next day. The client tells the nurse that she wants to wait until her family arrives later. Which nursing action is most appropriate?
   a. Ask the client to sign but inform her that she can change her mind.
   b. Ask the client if she has any questions you can answer.
   (c.) Tell the client to call you when her family arrives.
   d. Inform the physician.

   Rationale: The answer is (c). The family is an important social organization in many cultures. Being available when the family arrives is manifesting respect for the client's wishes and cultural sensitivity. Options (a), (b), and (d) do not address cultural sensitivity.

2. The nurse is taking care of a client who is scheduled for surgery today. The client asks the nurse to read a passage from the Bible to help her prepare herself for surgery. It is most appropriate for the nurse to:
   (a.) read the Bible passage.
   b. ask if someone on staff is the same religion as the client.
   c. kindly tell the client that nurses cannot get involved in religious issues.
   d. inquire whether the client would prefer that a religious person be called.

   Rationale: The answer is (a). Recognizing the spiritual needs of a client is viewing the client as a whole person with spiritual as well as physical needs. Options (b), (c), and (d) defer the needs of the patient to someone else.

3. The nurse is assigned to a client who believes that wearing a copper bracelet will relieve arthritic pain. In providing care for the client, it is most important for the nurse to:
   a. encourage the client to use anti-inflammatory medication.
   b. inform the client that copper bracelets have no proven medical value.
   c. address the pathophysiologic mechanisms associated with arthritis with the client.
   (d.) respect the beliefs associated with the copper bracelet by the client.

   Rationale: The answer is (d). Cultural beliefs play an important role in the healing process. This cultural belief does not interfere with the client's well-being. Options (a), (b), and (c) tend to minimize the client's belief.

INTRODUCTION TO FORMULATING A NURSING DIAGNOSIS

List the **five steps of the nursing process:**

1. ______________________
2. ______________________
3. ______________________
4. ______________________
5. ______________________

The **NANDA nursing diagnoses** are classified and formulated to address the client's health problems, which can be:

1. ______________________
2. ______________________
3. ______________________
4. ______________________

Circle the **words** that may be used to give specific meaning to the Nursing Diagnosis statement:

Related to
Increased
Ineffective
Well
Risk for
Acute
Impaired
Sign/Symptom
Due to
Possible

Case Study: The home health nurse makes the following observations and documents the following after visiting a 68-year-old male client: Lives alone, his only son lives 60 miles away, visits monthly, and calls weekly. The client stays indoors all day. His vision is poor and he is not able to drive.

Pertinent Terminology	Definition
NANDA	
Nursing process	
Assessment	
Nursing diagnosis	
Defining characteristics	
Planning	
Implementation	
Evaluation	
Etiology	

From the case study, **check off (✓) the nursing diagnosis** most appropriate for the client (use a nursing diagnosis book to validate your selection):

Nursing Diagnoses:
___ Coping, ineffective
___ Loneliness, risk for
___ Social isolation

List the **risk factors or defining characteristics** for the **nursing diagnosis** you selected:

______________________ ______________________ ______________________

______________________ ______________________

Further documentation by the home health nurse states: The client has lost 10 pounds since the last visit 2 weeks ago. He now is malnourished and lives on a limited income. He needs the services of a nutritionist and a community service that delivers meals to homebound individuals.

From the **further documentation** data, **check off (✓) the nursing diagnosis** most appropriate for the client:

Nursing Diagnoses:
___ Social isolation
___ Knowledge, deficient
___ Nutrition, imbalanced: less than body requirements

List the **current pertinent defining characteristics** for the nursing diagnosis you selected:

______________________ ______________________ ______________________

Interactive Activity: With a partner, review the following case studies and **identify** the **defining characteristics** that relate to the **nursing diagnosis** written next to each situation.

Case Study	Defining Characteristics
The client has a Stage II pressure ulcer on her right heel. She has been on bed rest and her right leg is elevated.	SKIN INTEGRITY, IMPAIRED ______________________
The client has oral lesions in his mouth caused by a treatment of chemotherapy. He complains of pain and his mouth is red.	ORAL MEMBRANES, IMPAIRED ______________________
The client is scheduled for surgery in the morning. She says that she is very scared because her grandmother died during surgery.	FEAR ______________________

FORMULATING A NURSING DIAGNOSIS

List the components of the:

One-part nursing diagnosis statement:

1. ______________________________

Two-part nursing diagnosis statement:

1. ______________________________
2. ______________________________

Three-part nursing diagnosis statement:

1. ______________________________
2. ______________________________
3. ______________________________

Place an "X" in the box that identifies the common errors made in the development of the nursing diagnosis statement:

- ☐ Using the NANDA diagnostic categories to identify the nursing diagnosis
- ☐ Using the medical diagnosis in the formulation of the nursing diagnosis
- ☐ Clustering the subjective/objective data
- ☐ Using signs and symptoms to write the nursing diagnosis statement
- ☐ Making legally inadvisable statements
- ☐ Misinterpreting the meaning of the subjective and objective data
- ☐ Being very specific in defining the etiology
- ☐ Using qualifying words in the diagnostic statement

Case Study: The client is to be scheduled for elective surgery. In preparation for the surgery, the office nurse takes the client's health history. The nurse documents that the client has recently been diagnosed with diabetes mellitus and was prescribed an antidiabetic pill to take every morning. The client tells the nurse that she stopped the "pill" 1 week ago because she was feeling better.

Pertinent Terminology	Definition
Nursing diagnosis	
Defining characteristics	
Risk factors	
Etiology	
Data cluster	

Use the **case study** to **cluster the subjective and objective data:**

Objective data: ____

____

Subjective data: ____

Use the data to complete the nursing diagnosis below with a **three-part statement** for the client:

Deficient knowledge: ____

____

Interactive Activity: With a partner, review the following case studies and (1) **list** the **defining characteristics**, (2) **identify the error** in the **nursing diagnosis** statement, and (3) **write a correct nursing diagnosis:**

Case Study

The client has been confused all morning. He has attempted to get out of bed and does not know who he is. His laboratory diagnostic studies indicate that he has a decreased serum sodium level. The nurse wrote the following nursing diagnosis:

Chronic confusion, r/t electrolyte imbalance

Defining Characteristics

____

____

Error(s)

____

____

____

____

____

Nursing Diagnosis

____

____

____

____

The client goes weekly to the outpatient clinic to have his blood pressure checked. He smokes one pack of cigarettes per day. His blood pressure is 146/88. His father died from heart disease at age 49 years, and his brother is recovering from a heart attack. The nurse writes the following nursing diagnosis:

Risk for heart attack r/t smoking and family history of heart disease

Defining Characteristics

____

____

Related Factors

____

____

____

____

Error(s)

____

____

____

____

____

Nursing Diagnosis

____

____

____

____

APPLYING CRITICAL THINKING SKILLS TO TEST QUESTIONS

INSTRUCTIONS: **Circle the one best answer for each test question.** Write your rationale for selecting the answer. To enhance your learning and test-taking skills, discuss your answer and rationale with a partner. The answer and the rationale can be found on the back of this page.

1. The nurse clusters the client's objective and subjective signs and symptoms primarily to:
   a. identify the nursing diagnosis.
   b. correlate with the medical diagnosis.
   c. validate the subjective complaints.
   d. work with "risk for" diagnoses.

   Rationale for your selection: ____
   ____
   ____
   ____
   ____
   ____

2. The following nursing diagnosis is found on the client rand: Hip fracture r/t fall. In evaluating the written diagnosis, the nurse correctly concludes that the diagnosis:
   a. is written appropriately.
   b. needs a modifier after the r/t statement.
   c. needs a modifier in the first part of the statement.
   d. is written inappropriately.

   Rationale for your selection: ____
   ____
   ____
   ____
   ____
   ____

3. The nurse admits an elderly client with the medical diagnosis of dehydration. In developing the nursing diagnoses, it is most important for the nurse to:
   a. establish nursing diagnoses that are based on the medical diagnosis.
   b. focus on nursing diagnoses that affect fluid balance.
   c. gather data to support actual nursing diagnoses.
   d. include actual and risk for diagnoses.

   Rationale for your selection: ____
   ____
   ____
   ____
   ____
   ____

ANSWER KEY FOR APPLYING CRITICAL THINKING SKILLS TO TEST QUESTIONS

HELPFUL HINTS: Read all test questions carefully. Identify key words in the question that will guide you in answering the question. In these test questions the **key words** to consider are **"primarily," "correctly concludes,"** and **"most important."** Compare your rationale with the one in the test question.

1. The nurse clusters the client's objective and subjective signs and symptoms primarily to
   (a.) identify the nursing diagnosis.
   b. correlate with the medical diagnosis.
   c. validate the subjective complaints.
   d. work with "risk for" diagnoses.

   Rationale: The answer is (a). Clustering the data helps the nurse to identify the defining characteristic that led to the formulation of a nursing diagnosis. Options (b) and (c) do not apply, and option (d) addresses only "risk for" diagnoses.

2. The following nursing diagnosis is found on the client rand: Hip fracture r/t fall. In evaluating the written diagnosis, the nurse correctly concludes that the diagnosis:
   a. is written appropriately.
   b. needs a modifier after the r/t statement.
   c. needs a modifier in the first part of the statement.
   (d.) is written inappropriately.

   Rationale: The answer is (d). Hip fracture is a medical diagnosis. The nurse needs to identify the defining characteristics and then select the appropriate nursing diagnosis. Options (a), (b), and (c) do not apply to this example.

3. The nurse admits an elderly client with the medical diagnosis of dehydration. In developing the nursing diagnoses, it is most important for the nurse to:
   a. establish nursing diagnoses that are based on the medical diagnosis.
   b. focus on nursing diagnoses that affect fluid balance.
   c. gather data to support actual nursing diagnoses.
   (d.) include actual and "risk for" diagnoses.

   Rationale: The answer is (d). Nursing includes the development of actual nursing diagnoses and any "risk for" diagnoses to provide total, safe care to the client. Option (a) is not correct and options (b) and (c) do not include the monitoring of possible complications.

ASSESSMENT OF THE ELDERLY PATIENT

List the **interventions** that would assist in communicating with an elderly patient who has hearing loss related to the aging process:

1. ______________________
2. ______________________
3. ______________________
4. ______________________
5. ______________________
6. ______________________

List the **interventions** that would assist an elderly patient who has vision problems related to the aging process:

1. ______________________
2. ______________________
3. ______________________
4. ______________________
5. ______________________
6. ______________________

Mark an "X" in the appropriate column that identifies the effects of aging on the following:

	Decreased	Increased
Sensory perception	☐	☐
Visual acuity	☐	☐
Gag reflex	☐	☐
Skin tissue elasticity	☐	☐
Body temperature	☐	☐
Cardiac output	☐	☐
RBC production	☐	☐
Plasma viscosity	☐	☐
Lung capacity	☐	☐
Residual urine	☐	☐

Case Study: The following information has been given to a group of students regarding the assessment of an elderly patient: Responds slowly but appropriately to all questions. Skin warm, dry, thin, and flaky. Skin turgor >3 sec. Capillary refill >3 sec. Respirations short and shallow, lung sounds with bilateral crackles. 50% intake, states food is very bland. BM this morning moderate amount formed hard stool. Bilateral lower extremities with 1+ pitting edema. Toenails yellowish, thick. Vital signs T 99° F, P 84, R 16, BP 160/80.

Pertinent Terminology	Definition
Arcus senilis	
Edema	
Pitting edema	
Kyphosis	
Presbycusis	
Presbyopia	
Turgor	

Use the information from the case study below to mark an "X" on the data that are representative of the normal effects of the aging process:

___ Responds slowly, but appropriately to all questions
___ Skin warm, dry, thin, and flaky
___ Skin turgor >3 sec; capillary refill >3 sec
___ Respirations short and shallow, lung sounds with bilateral crackles
___ 50% intake, states food is very bland
___ BM this morning formed hard stool
___ Bilateral lower extremities with 1+ pitting edema
___ Toenails yellowish, thick
___ Vital signs T 99° F, P 84, R 16, BP 160/80

Interactive Activity: With a partner, use the information provided to (1) **underline** the assessment data that represent the **effects of the normal aging process** and (2) **select** the NANDA nursing diagnosis most appropriate for the situation:

Assessment Data	Nursing Diagnosis
Wife in to see patient, states that husband is confused this morning, does not know that he is in the hospital. Further patient assessment, PERRL, whitish ring noted around the margins of the iris, uses glasses. Mouth dry, wears upper dentures.	☐ Disturbed thought processes ☐ Impaired oral mucous membrane ☐ Acute confusion ☐ Impaired memory
Skin pale, translucent. Lower extremities thin, pedal pulses weak, palpable. States has loss of a small amount of urine when coughs. Shortness of breath, R 28, mouth breathing. Abdomen round, soft, nontender. Temp. 96.8° F.	☐ Functional urinary incontinence ☐ Hypothermia ☐ Ineffective tissue perfusion ☐ Ineffective breathing pattern
Transfers independently out of bed, complained of dizziness when coming to a standing position, gait slow. Anterior-posterior diameter of chest increased. Soft diet, intake 70%.	☐ Impaired physical mobility ☐ Risk for injury ☐ Ineffective health maintenance ☐ Imbalanced nutrition: less than body requirements

CARING FOR THE SURGICAL PATIENT

List the **two major** types of anesthesia:

1. ______________________________
2. ______________________________

List the **types of regional anesthesia**:

1. ______________________________
2. ______________________________
3. ______________________________
4. ______________________________
5. ______________________________

Identify in which of the perioperative phases (**preoperative, intraoperative, postoperative**) the following interventions would be started:

	Pre	Intra	Post
Use of incentive spirometer	☐	☐	☐
Coughing and deep breathing	☐	☐	☐
Splinting of surgical site	☐	☐	☐
Prepping surgical site	☐	☐	☐
Changing the surgical dressing	☐	☐	☐
Leg exercises	☐	☐	☐
Pain management	☐	☐	☐
Discharge instructions	☐	☐	☐

Case Study: A female patient is admitted for a total abdominal hysterectomy this morning. She is 52 years old and obese. Her medical history indicates that she stopped smoking 5 years ago. Both parents are deceased. Mother died at the age of 88 years and father died from a heart attack at the age of 62. The client's vital signs are: T 97.8° F, P 76, R 18, BP 164/92. The following laboratory studies were done: CBC, PT, serum electrolytes of Na^+, K^+, serum FBG, BUN, and creatinine. The UA, chest x-ray report, and ECG report are in the chart.

Pertinent Terminology	Definition
General anesthesia	______________________________
Regional anesthesia	______________________________
Thrombophlebitis	______________________________
Atelectasis	______________________________
Paralytic ileus	______________________________
PCA	______________________________
Sequential stockings	______________________________

From the case study, **list** the factors that increase the patient's risk of postoperative complications:

______________________ ______________________

______________________ ______________________

Interactive Activity: With a partner, use the follow-up case study to (1) **identify** which medical order the nurse would do **first** and (2) **list the priority nursing interventions** the nurse would **independently perform** and provide a **rationale** for each intervention:

Follow-up case study: The patient returns from the postanesthesia room sleepy but easily arousable. The physician writes the following postoperative orders:

NPO—May have sips of water in the AM
IV—Dextrose 5/0.9% Normal Saline infuse at 100 mL/hr
Ambulate this evening
VS q30 min for first hour, then q1h × 2 hr, then q4h
Incentive spirometer q1h while awake
PCA—Morphine sulfate set at 1 mg/6 min (per patient demand not to exceed 30 mg/4 hr)
Antiembolic stockings and sequential stockings to legs continuously
Indwelling urinary catheter to gravity—remove in AM

First Medical Orders to Implement	Rationale
1. ______________________	______________________

Priority Independent Nursing Interventions	Rationale
1. ______________________	______________________
2. ______________________	______________________
3. ______________________	______________________
4. ______________________	______________________
5. ______________________	______________________
6. ______________________	______________________
7. ______________________	______________________

APPLYING CRITICAL THINKING SKILLS TO TEST QUESTIONS

INSTRUCTIONS: Circle the one best answer for each test question. Write your rationale for selecting the answer. To enhance your learning and test-taking skills, discuss your answer and rationale with a partner. The answer and the rationale can be found on the back of this page.

1. The client is transferred to the surgical unit from the postanesthesia room after having abdominal surgery. There is a J-P drainage device in place. Which of the following reported findings on transfer requires immediate follow-up?
   a. Abdominal dressing reinforced in the recovery room
   b. R 14, P 86, BP 126/90, lethargic but responds to touch
   c. Bowel sounds absent in all quadrants
   d. J-P compressed with 10 mL reddish drainage

   Rationale for your selection: ____
   ____
   ____
   ____
   ____
   ____

2. Which of the following client statements is correct in describing the appropriate use of the incentive spirometer?
   a. "I will first inhale then blow into the mouthpiece."
   b. "I will put the mouthpiece in my mouth and blow into the mouthpiece."
   c. "I will put the mouthpiece in my mouth and then inhale slowly."
   d. "I will put the mouthpiece in my mouth, inhale, and hold for 5 seconds."

   Rationale for your selection: ____
   ____
   ____
   ____
   ____
   ____

3. The nurse is preparing a client for emergency surgery. Before surgery, it is most important for the nurse to ensure that the:
   a. preop checklist is completed.
   b. preop medications are documented.
   c. lab results are in the chart.
   d. surgical consent is signed.

   Rationale for your selection: ____
   ____
   ____
   ____
   ____
   ____

ANSWER KEY FOR APPLYING CRITICAL THINKING SKILLS TO TEST QUESTIONS

HELPFUL HINTS: Read all test questions carefully. Identify key words in the question that will guide you in answering the question. In these test questions the **key words** to consider are **"immediate,"** **"correct,"** and **"most important."** Compare your rationale with the one in the test question.

1. The client is transferred to the surgical unit from the postanesthesia room after having abdominal surgery. There is a J-P drainage device in place. Which of the following reported findings on transfer requires immediate follow-up?
   (a.) Abdominal dressing reinforced in the recovery room
   b. R 14, P 86, BP 126/90, lethargic but responds to touch
   c. Bowel sounds absent in all quadrants
   d. J-P compressed with 10 mL reddish drainage

   Rationale: The answer is (a). Reinforcement of the surgical dressing indicates excessive drainage; this should be carefully monitored. Option (b) indicates vital signs within normal limits, and options (c) and (d) are expected findings for a client who has had abdominal surgery.

2. Which of the following client statements is correct in describing the appropriate use of the incentive spirometer?
   a. "I will first inhale then blow into the mouthpiece."
   b. "I will put the mouthpiece in my mouth and blow into the mouthpiece."
   (c.) "I will put the mouthpiece in my mouth and then inhale slowly."
   d. "I will put the mouthpiece in my mouth, inhale, and hold for 5 seconds."

   Rationale: The answer is (c). This describes the procedure appropriately. Options (a) and (b) do not describe the procedure correctly, and option (d) is partially correct but the client does not need to hold for 5 seconds.

3. The nurse is preparing a client for emergency surgery. Before surgery, it is most important for the nurse to ensure that the:
   a. preop checklist is completed.
   b. preop medications are documented.
   c. lab results are in the chart.
   (d.) surgical consent is signed.

   Rationale: The answer is (d). Although the physician is responsible for obtaining the client's signature, it is most important for the nurse to ensure that it has been signed. Options (a), (b), and (c) are important but are not the most important.

WOUND ASSESSMENT

List the **types of wounds:**

1. ______________________________
2. ______________________________

List the **types of wound drainage** systems:

1. ______________________________
2. ______________________________
3. ______________________________

Match the **wound classifications and wound drainage terminology** with the appropriate description or characteristics:

1. Laceration	____	Thin, clear watery secretion
2. Contusion	____	Containing pus
3. Penetrating	____	Open cut made with a knife/scalpel
4. Abrasion	____	Containing RBCs
5. Incision	____	Irregular wound tear; jagged edges
6. Serosangineous	____	Entering into the tissues/body cavity
7. Serous	____	Closed wound; with pain, swelling, and discoloration
8. Sangineous	____	Red, watery secretion
9. Purulent	____	A scraping away of the skin surface

Case Study: Mr. J, 26 years old, received a stab wound to his abdomen and was taken to the emergency department. He underwent emergency surgery. He has an IV, nasogastric tube to continuous low wall suction, and one Jackson-Pratt on the right upper quadrant and another on the left lower quadrant of the abdomen. He has a closed abdominal wound and the dressing is clean and dry as he is taken to the surgical unit at 0800.

Pertinent Terminology	Definition
Primary intention	
Tertiary intention	
Secondary intention	
Granulation tissue	
Inflammatory phase	
Proliferation phase	
Maturation phase	
Dehiscence	
Evisceration	

Use the case study to **check off** (✓) all the factors that apply to Mr. J:

- ☐ High risk for infection
- ☐ Healing by secondary intention
- ☐ J-P will aid in the healing process
- ☐ Postop pain should initially increase
- ☐ J-P drainage should progressively decrease
- ☐ Slight redness around incision first day

Three hours after arriving on the surgical unit, the nurse took the vital signs and noted that Mr. J's surgical dressing has two abd pads and the dressing is currently saturated with sangineous drainage. The nurse lightly palpated the abdomen.

Implement the appropriate nursing interventions on the abdominal surgical dressing:

Abdominal Surgical Dressing

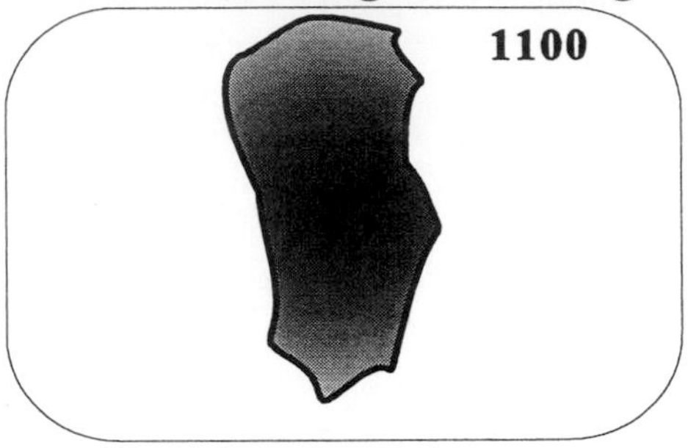

Select the nurse's documentation that demonstrates appropriate assessment:

___ Abdominal dressing with large amount of red drainage, abdomen tender, T 100.4° F

___ Abdominal dressing covered with pink reddish drainage, abdomen tender, no bowel sounds, P 88, BP 136/86

___ Abdominal dressing saturated with red drainage, abdomen tender, reinforced, P 88, BP 136/86

Interactive Activity: With a partner, use the **statements** below to (1) **check** (✓) **whether the statement is correct or incorrect and** (2) **provide a rationale for your selection.**

Statements	Correct/Incorrect	Rationale
1. Wound drainage devices need to be emptied once a shift.	☐ Correct ☐ Incorrect	______ ______
2. Wound drainage devices need to be compressed to function.	☐ Correct ☐ Incorrect	______ ______
3. Assessment of the wound should be done once a day.	☐ Correct ☐ Incorrect	______ ______
4. Wound description does not need to include wound measurement.	☐ Correct ☐ Incorrect	______ ______
5. Wound evisceration requires the application of sterile dry gauze.	☐ Correct ☐ Incorrect	______ ______

APPLYING CRITICAL THINKING SKILLS TO TEST QUESTIONS

INSTRUCTIONS: Circle the one best answer for each test question. Write your rationale for selecting the answer. To enhance your learning and test-taking skills, discuss your answer and rationale with a partner. The answer and the rationale can be found on the back of this page.

1. An elderly client is being discharged after abdominal surgery. The staples were removed on the third day after surgery and a gauze dressing was applied. The client tells the nurse that as he was standing up he heard a pop coming from his abdomen. Which nursing intervention is of priority?
   a. Fully assess the neurologic status of the client.
   b. Auscultate the bowel sounds.
   c. Assess the surgical site.
   d. Palpate the abdomen.

   Rationale for your selection: ______________________________

2. On the second day after surgery, the nurse assesses a surgical wound and documents the following, "Surgical incision with stitches intact, erythema noted on surrounding skin around surgical incision, edges well approximated." Based on this documentation, the nurse most accurately assessed that the surgical wound:
   a. is healing without complications.
   b. is beginning to show signs of complications.
   c. needs to be assessed by the physician.
   d. will take longer to heal.

   Rationale for your selection: ______________________________

3. The physician orders the following dressing changes for an elderly client who has an open wound on the sacrum: "Apply hydrocolloid dressing on the wound. Change dressing every 3 days." The primary purpose of the dressing is to:
   a. enhance healing by primary intention.
   b. absorb wound drainage.
   c. provide moisture to the area.
   d. protect the wound from additional pressure.

   Rationale for your selection: ______________________________

ANSWER KEY FOR APPLYING CRITICAL THINKING SKILLS TO TEST QUESTIONS

HELPFUL HINTS: Read all test questions carefully. Identify key words in the question that will guide you in answering the question. In these test questions the **key words** to consider are **"priority," "most accurately,"** and **"primary purpose."** Compare your rationale with the one found for each question.

1. An elderly client is being discharged after abdominal surgery. The staples were removed on the third day after surgery and a gauze dressing was applied. The client tells the nurse that as he was standing up he heard a pop coming from his abdomen. Which nursing intervention is of priority?
   a. Fully assess the neurologic status of the client.
   b. Auscultate the bowel sounds.
   (c.) Assess the surgical site.
   d. Palpate the abdomen.

   Rationale: The answer is (c). Wound dehiscence is a possible complication. Clients may not have any pain. With option (a) not enough data are present to suggest that a full neurologic assessment is warranted, and options (b) and (d) should be done after inspection.

2. On the second day after surgery, the nurse assesses a surgical wound and documents the following, "Surgical incision with stitches intact, erythema noted on surrounding skin around surgical incision, edges well approximated." Based on this documentation, the nurse most accurately assessed that the surgical wound:
   (a.) is healing without complications.
   b. is beginning to show signs of complications.
   c. needs to be assessed by the physician.
   d. will take longer to heal.

   Rationale: The answer is (a). Documentation describes the normal healing process of a second postoperative day surgical wound. Options (b), (c), and (d) are not appropriate at this time.

3. The physician orders the following dressing changes for an elderly client who has an open wound on the sacrum: "Apply hydrocolloid dressing on the wound. Change dressing every 3 days." The primary purpose of the dressing is to:
   a. enhance healing by primary intention.
   (b.) absorb wound drainage.
   c. provide moisture to the area.
   d. protect the wound from additional pressure.

   Rationale: The answer is (b). Hydrocolloid dressings help to remove exudates from a wound. Option (a) is incorrect because the wound will heal by secondary intention; options (c) and (d) are not the primary purpose for applying this dressing.

WOUND DRESSINGS

List the **types of wound dressings:**

1. ______________________________
2. ______________________________
3. ______________________________
4. ______________________________
5. ______________________________

Alginate: ______________________________
____

Hydrogel: ______________________________
____
____
____

Hydrocolloid: ______________________________
____
____
____
____

Transparent: ______________________________
____
____
____

Wet-dry gauze dressing: ______________________________
____

Case Study: Mr. Y, 78 years old, has been in the acute care setting for 2 months. He was admitted with a fractured left hip, anorexia, and weight loss. He has a Stage IV pressure ulcer on the sacrum with undermining at 12 o'clock and a Stage II pressure ulcer of the right heel. The physician writes the following orders: irrigate the sacral wound daily with normal saline solution. Pack wound with a wet-dry dressing with normal saline solution every shift. Apply a hydrocolloid dressing to the right heel every 3 days.

Pertinent Terminology	Definition
Debridement	
Exudate	
Macerate	
Mechanical debridement	
Wound irrigation	
Wet-dry	

The nurse is preparing to irrigate and change the dressing of the sacral wound. Select all the statements that apply to the wound irrigation and to the application of the wet-dry dressing.

Wound Irrigation

- ☐ Clean the wound bed with iodine
- ☐ Use a 35-mL syringe
- ☐ Irrigate with 0.9% normal saline solution
- ☐ Use a 3-mL syringe with a 22-gauge needle
- ☐ Attach an 18-gauge angiocath to the irrigating syringe

Sacral Wet-Dry Dressing

- ☐ Lightly pack the moist gauze into the wound bed
- ☐ Pack the dry dressing into the wound first
- ☐ Lightly pack the area of undermining with the moist dressing
- ☐ Lightly pack the area of undermining with the dry dressing
- ☐ Allow the moist dressing to cover the outside surface of the skin

The nurse writes the following data on the clinical worksheet:

Sacral wound
0900 Size 3.5 cm by 4.0 cm, irregular margins. Pressure ulcer 2.5 cm deep. Slough at margins. Tan-colored drainage moderate amount. Checked for undermining. 1.2 cm undermining at 12 o'clock. Old dressing removed. Wet-dry dressing applied. Irrigated with saline solution with a large syringe. Medicated with analgesic 30 minutes prior to procedure. Tolerated well.

Right heel wound
0900 Hydrocolloid dressing changed on right heel. No changes from the previous dressing change 3 days ago.

Interactive Activity: With a partner, discuss the wound assessment observations made by the nurse. For the **sacral wound**—rewrite the assessment observations in the space provided.

For the **right heel wound**—identify why the documentation made by the nurse is *not* appropriate.

THE PATIENT WITH FLUID AND ELECTROLYTE IMBALANCE

List the **adult normal values** for the following electrolytes:

1. Sodium (Na^+) = ____________________
2. Potassium (K^+) = ____________________
3. Chloride (Cl^-) = ____________________
4. Calcium (Ca^{++}) = ____________________
5. Phosphate (PO_4^-) = ____________________
6. Magnesium (Mg^{++}) = ____________________

Write in the appropriate medical terminology for the serum laboratory values below:

Mg^{++} 3.5 mg/dl = ____________________

K^+ 2.5 mEq/L = ____________________

Cl^- 90 mEq/L = ____________________

Na^+ 132 mEq/L = ____________________

Ca^{++} 8.5 mg/dL = ____________________

PO_4^- 5.1 mg/dL = ____________________

Case Study: A 36-year-old client was admitted with gastroenteritis. He has been vomiting and having severe diarrhea for 2 days. He is very weak. The current laboratory results are Na^+ 128 mEq/L, K^+ 2.8 mEq/L, Cl^- 90 mEq/L. The physician orders IV of 0.9% normal saline solution at 100 mL/hr, NPO, and I & O.

Pertinent Terminology	Definition
Sodium (Na^+)	
Potassium (K^+)	
Chloride (Cl^-)	
Calcium (Ca^{++})	
Phosphate (PO_4^-)	
Magnesium (Mg^{++})	
Third space syndrome	
Edema	
Pitting edema	

From the case study, identify the abnormal laboratory results. List the **major clinical signs or symptoms** that you would assess with each abnormal value:

____________________ = ____
____
____

____________________ = ____
____
____

____________________ = ____
____
____

Follow-up case study: The client's vomiting and diarrhea has begun to subside in the evening and the MD has ordered a clear liquid diet. The client's **24-hour I & O** for the day is charted below:

24-Hour Intake/Output Record

IV	=	2400	Emesis	=	950
Oral	=	120	Diarrhea	=	900
			Urine	=	750
		2520 mL			2600 mL

On the basis of the case study and Intake and Output Record, **select** the most appropriate **NANDA nursing diagnoses** for the client:

___ Excess fluid volume
___ Diarrhea
___ Imbalanced nutrition: Less than body requirements
___ Deficient fluid volume
___ Impaired skin integrity
___ Risk for injury

Interactive Activity: With a partner, read the case study below and write a rationale for each of the nursing interventions listed:

Case Study	Nursing Interventions	Rationale
Ms. M was admitted with heart failure. The nursing diagnosis of "Fluid volume excess r/t noncompliance to dietary Na^+ restriction" is listed in her NCP. Digoxin 0.25 mg qAM po, furosemide 40 mg qAM po, and K-dur 10 mEq po tid are her medications.	Weigh daily	____________
	Monitor I & O	____________
	Take apical pulse	____________
	Assess skin	____________
	Assess lungs	____________
	✓ Neck veins	____________

ELIMINATION—URINARY

List the **factors** that affect bladder elimination:

1. ______
2. ______
3. ______
4. ______
5. ______
6. ______
7. ______
8. ______
9. ______

Use the diagrams to **select** the appropriate size of the indwelling catheter for the female and male patient. **Draw a line** on the catheter at the anticipated length of insertion.

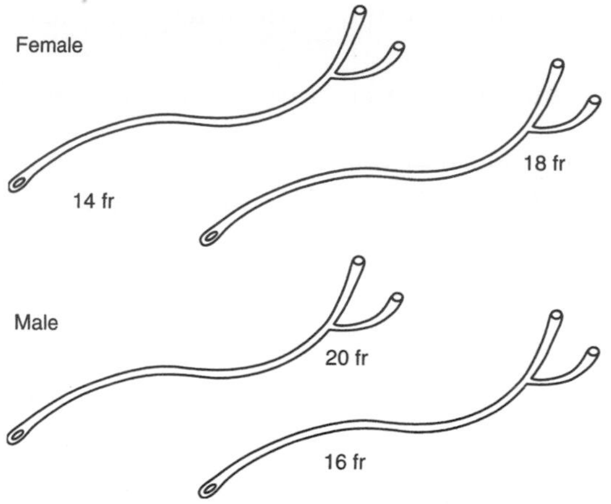

Case Study: Mrs. S, a 42-year-old woman, had abdominal surgery 2 days ago. She has an IV infusing into her left forearm, an indwelling urinary catheter (Foley), and she has a temperature of 100.4° F this evening. The physician orders the indwelling catheter to be removed in the AM.

Pertinent Terminology	Definition
UA	
Nocturia	
Hematuria	
Dysuria	
Oliguria	
Anuria	
Urinary incontinence	
Residual urine	
Midstream UA	
Void	
Indwelling catheter	
Condom catheter	

Using the information in the case study, the nurse gathers more information and documents on Mrs. S's chart. **Select the statement** below that describes a thorough observation of the urinary system:

1. Indwelling catheter patent to gravity, taking fluids liberally
2. Indwelling catheter to gravity, draining cloudy pale yellow urine
3. Indwelling catheter patent to gravity, output 75 mL
4. Indwelling catheter patent, draining freely; abdomen without distention

The next morning, the nurse prepares to remove the indwelling catheter. Identify the equipment the nurse needs to gather to properly remove the catheter.

____

The indwelling catheter is removed at 0800. The nurse knows that Mrs. S should void within _________ hours after removal of the catheter.

Interactive Activity: With a partner, **select the NANDA nursing diagnosis** that is most appropriate to the case studies below that describe the complications Mrs. S had after removal of the indwelling catheter.

NANDA nursing diagnosis: (1) Incontinence, stress urinary (2) Urinary retention (3) Urinary elimination, impaired (4) Infection, risk for

Case Study	Nursing Diagnosis
Mrs. S is unable to void 8 hours after removal of the indwelling catheter. She has abdominal discomfort, a sensation of fullness, and frequent dribbling.	______________
Mrs. S is catheterized for residual urine and 700 mL of urine are drained from the bladder. An indwelling catheter is left in place again.	______________
The following day the catheter is removed. Mrs. S is able to void without any further problems that day. The next day she complains of dysuria and hematuria when she voids.	______________
Mrs. S is started on an antibiotic. She notices that the dysuria and hematuria are no longer present. However, she tells you that she has a history of losing urine when she coughs or sneezes.	______________

APPLYING CRITICAL THINKING SKILLS TO TEST QUESTIONS

INSTRUCTIONS: **Circle the one best answer for each test question.** Write your rationale for selecting the answer. To enhance your learning and test-taking skills, discuss your answer and rationale with a partner. The answer and the rationale can be found on the back of this page.

1. The physician writes the following order on admission for an adult female patient, "Insert Foley catheter stat." It is most appropriate for the nurse to initially insert a:
   a. 14 Fr catheter.
   b. 16 Fr catheter.
   c. 20 Fr catheter.
   d. 22 Fr catheter.

   Rationale for your selection: ____
   ____
   ____
   ____
   ____
   ____

2. The nurse is caring for a client who has a urinary catheter. To accurately assess the urine color, it is most important for the nurse to:
   a. look at the color and amount of urine in the drainage bag.
   b. draw 1 to 2 mL of urine from the catheter port.
   c. look at the color of the urine in the drainage tube.
   d. review the color of the urine documented by the previous shift.

   Rationale for your selection: ____
   ____
   ____
   ____
   ____
   ____

3. The physician writes the following order: "I & O cath for residual this AM." Which statement, given to a nursing assistant by the nurse, is most helpful for implementing this order?
   a. "Let me know when the client wants to void."
   b. "Let me know as soon as the client voids."
   c. "Push fluids this morning."
   d. "Record how much the client voids this morning."

   Rationale for your selection: ____
   ____
   ____
   ____
   ____
   ____

ANSWER KEY FOR APPLYING CRITICAL THINKING SKILLS TO TEST QUESTIONS

HELPFUL HINTS: Read all test questions carefully. Identify key words in the question that will guide you in answering the question. In these test questions the **key words** to consider are **"most appropriate," "accurately assess," "most important,"** and **"most helpful."** Compare your rationale with the one in the test question.

1. The physician writes the following order on admission for an adult female patient, "Insert Foley catheter stat." It is most appropriate for the nurse to initially insert a:
   (a.) 14 Fr catheter.
   b. 16 Fr catheter.
   c. 20 Fr catheter.
   d. 22 Fr catheter.

   Rationale: The answer is (a). The nurse will insert the smallest catheter to avoid trauma and unnecessary dilation of the urethra. Option (b) can be used if a 14 Fr is not available. Options (c) and (d) are too large in diameter for a routine catheterization.

2. The nurse is caring for a client who has a urinary catheter. To accurately assess the urine color, it is most important for the nurse to:
   a. look at the color and amount of urine in the drainage bag.
   b. draw 1 to 2 mL of urine from the catheter port.
   (c.) look at the color of the urine in the drainage tube.
   d. review the color of the urine documented by the previous shift.

   Rationale: The answer is (c). The color of the urine is best noted in the drainage tube because the tube contains the most recent urine coming from the bladder. Option (b) is used to obtain a urine specimen, option (a) is not the best since urine collecting in the bag may look darker, and option (d) does not provide the most current assessment of the urine.

3. The physician writes the following order: "I & O cath for residual this AM." Which statement, given to a nursing assistant by the nurse, is most helpful for implementing this order?
   a. "Let me know when the client wants to void."
   (b.) "Let me know as soon as the client voids."
   c. "Push fluids this morning."
   d. "Record how much the client voids this morning."

   Rationale: The answer is (b). Catheterizing for residual requires that the procedure be implemented as soon as the client voids. This will provide information as to the amount of urine left in the bladder after the client has voided. Options (a), (c), and (d) do not address the directions needed for implementing the order.

ELIMINATION—BOWEL

List the **factors** that affect bowel elimination:

1. ______________________________
2. ______________________________
3. ______________________________
4. ______________________________
5. ______________________________
6. ______________________________
7. ______________________________

Use the diagram to identify the location and placement of the stethoscope when listening for bowel sounds. Draw a circle at each location.

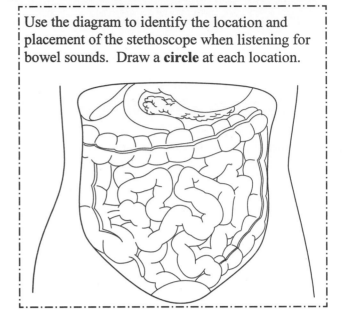

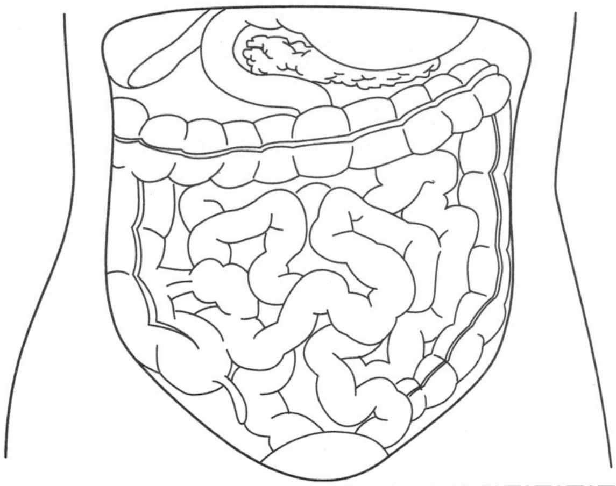

Case Study: The physician writes the following on the history and physical form after examining a 55-year-old client, Mr. M: "Complains of cramping abdominal pain, borborygmi, 5-6 dark brown semiliquid BMs/day for several days. Last bowel movement this AM. Indicates no changes in diet intake. Denies melena, constipation, nausea, or vomiting." The MD orders an endoscopy, barium enema, and stool for occult blood.

Pertinent Terminology	Definition
Bowel sounds	
Flatus	
Constipation	
Diarrhea	
Occult blood	
Melena	
Enema	
Fecal impaction	
Borborygmi	
Endoscopy	
Barium enema	

Using the information identified in the history and physical, identify the questions that the nurse could ask Mr. M to **assess** the bowel pattern changes that he is currently experiencing:

1. Complains of cramping abdominal pain, borborygmi

   Question: ______________________________

2. 5-6 dark brown semiliquid BMs/day for several days

   Question: ______________________________

3. Indicates no changes in diet intake

   Question: ______________________________

4. Denies melena, constipation, nausea, or vomiting

   Question: ______________________________

   ____

5. Last bowel movement this AM

   Question: ______________________________

Write two questions that would be useful in further assessing Mr. M's bowel function:

1. ______________________________

2. ______________________________

Discuss how these questions contribute to the assessment.

Interactive Activity: With a partner, select the **NANDA nursing diagnosis** that best applies to each of the case scenarios below:

NANDA nursing diagnosis:	(1) Constipation, perceived	(2) Diarrhea
	(3) Constipation (colonic)	(4) Bowel incontinence

Case Study	**Nursing Diagnosis**
The client takes a mild laxative every night since his retirement 1 year ago. He believes that his change in activity will cause him bowel problems.	______________
The client was in a car accident 1 month ago in which she sustained a neuromuscular back injury. While hospitalized she was having involuntary frequent loose BMs.	______________
The nursing diagnosis for Mr. M in the case study is:	______________

GENERAL NUTRITION

List the **four basic diets** commonly encountered in the clinical setting (exclude the special diets):

1. ____________________
2. ____________________
3. ____________________
4. ____________________

List the most common methods of providing enteral nutrition:

1. ____________________
2. ____________________
3. ____________________
4. ____________________

Draw a line to connect the following **foods** with the appropriate **common therapeutic diets** encountered in the clinical setting:

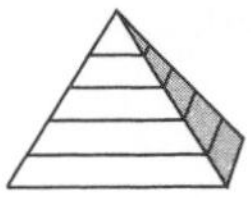

Clear Liquid

Ice cream
Carbonated beverages
Broth fat-free
Cooked vegetables
Cream of rice
Puddings
Smooth peanut butter
Clear fruit juices
Bananas
Custard
Sherbet
Eggs

Soft

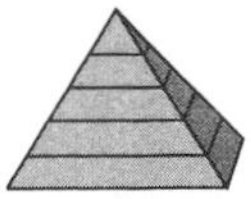

Full Liquid

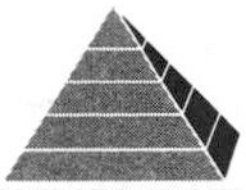

Case Study: A 68-year-old male client had a cerebral vascular accident 2 weeks ago. He has right-sided hemiplegia. The nursing care rand indicates that the client is on a soft pureed diet with thickened liquids and is on intake and output.

Pertinent Terminology	Definition
Regular diet	
Soft diet	
Full liquid	
Clear liquid	
Pureed	
Enteral nutrition	
Gastric gavage	
Nasogastric tube	
PEG	
Jejunostomy tube	

Use the information from the case study to **mark an** "X" on the most appropriate feeding guidelines for the client who has right-sided hemiplegia:

Feeding Guidelines

- ☐ Give water frequently with the food
- ☐ Check right cheek for "pocketing"
- ☐ Place in semi-Fowler's position
- ☐ Allow family to feed Mr. G
- ☐ Place in high Fowler's position
- ☐ Give thickened juices
- ☐ Provide finger foods
- ☐ Lie flat after feeding

Interactive Activity: With a partner, use the case studies related to the client. For each situation, **prioritize the NANDA nursing diagnosis,** **#1** = Priority, **#2** = Important, and **#3** = Need to monitor.

Case Study	NANDA Nursing Diagnosis
The client's intake for last 24 hr = 1250 mL and his output = 725 mL. He is fatigued and needs to be reminded to drink and eat. His skin is dry and flaky. Skin turgor—tenting. Oral mucous membranes dry, teeth missing. Urine color is dark yellow.	___ Deficient fluid volume r/t decreased fluid intake secondary to fatigue ___ Risk for impaired oral mucous membranes r/t insufficient intake of fluids ___ Risk for impaired skin integrity r/t dry, thin skin secondary to aging
The client began to cough forcefully while being fed. The feeding was stopped and the MD ordered for him to be NPO. The client has lost 3 pounds in 1 week. He has an IV of D5W infusing at 75 mL/hr. It is difficult to get him out of bed because he is weak and does not assist with the transfer.	___ Imbalanced nutrition r/t weakness, fatigue, and NPO status ___ Risk for aspiration r/t impaired swallowing ___ Risk for impaired skin integrity r/t prolonged bed rest

GASTROINTESTINAL TRACT

List the structures in the gastrointestinal tract involved with the digestion and absorption of food:

1. ______________________
2. ______________________
3. ______________________
4. ______________________
5. ______________________

Use the diagram to **identify the quadrants** (RLQ, RUQ, LLQ, LUQ) and the **anatomical regions of the abdomen** (Right and Left Lumbar, Right and Left Inguinal, Umbilical, Epigastric, Suprapubic, and Right and Left Hypochondriac)

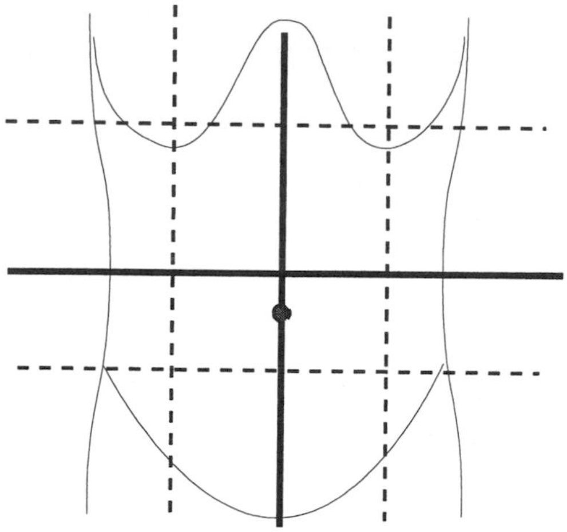

Modified from Black JM, Hawks JH, Keene AM: *Medical-surgical nursing: clinical management for positive outcomes*, ed 8, St. Louis, 2009, WB Saunders.

Case Study: Mrs. T is a 55-year-old woman who was admitted to the hospital with complaints of diarrhea for the past 10 days. She states that she has abdominal cramping and at times passes bloody stools. She is scheduled for a colonoscopy at 10:00 AM today.

Pertinent Terminology	Definition
Duodenum	
Jejunum	
Ileum	
Cecum	
Colon	
Rectum	
Polyp	

Use the case study to **check off (✓) all the nursing interventions and physician's orders** that you would associate with the preparation of Mrs. T for the colonoscopy procedure.

- ☐ NPO for procedure
- ☐ GoLytely will be given for stool evacuation
- ☐ Monitor for abdominal pain and bleeding after the procedure
- ☐ Consent is necessary
- ☐ May have a clear liquid breakfast
- ☐ Requires general anesthesia

Match the gastrointestinal diagnostic tests with the appropriate definitions:

Diagnostic test		Definitions
1. Colonoscopy	___	Visualization of the rectum and sigmoid
2. Endoscopy	___	Visualization from anus to cecum
3. Sigmoidoscopy	___	Visualization of esophagus, stomach, and small bowel
4. Barium swallow	___	Visualization of interior organs and structures using a fiberoptic instrument

Interactive Activity: With a partner, use the diagram to:

1. Identify the segments of the large intestine.
2. Follow the path of the colonoscopy procedure.
3. Identify the consistency of the stool as it moves through the intestinal tract (mushy, semiliquid, and solid).

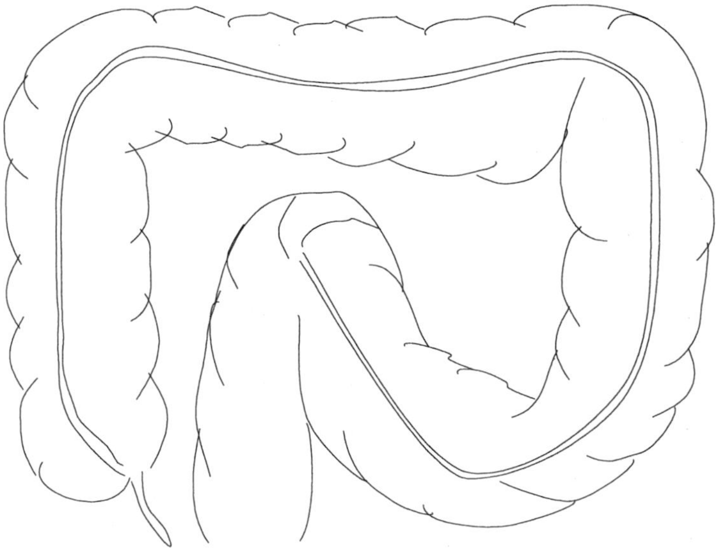

APPLYING CRITICAL THINKING SKILLS TO TEST QUESTIONS

INSTRUCTIONS: Circle the one best answer for each test question. Write your rationale for selecting the answer. To enhance your learning and test-taking skills, discuss your answer and rationale with a partner. The answer and the rationale can be found on the back of this page.

1. The client is scheduled for a UGI endoscopy. Which statement is correct in providing the client with information about this endoscopic procedure?
   a. "A tube will be passed from your nose into your stomach."
   b. "The tube is small, is very flexible, and has a light at the end."
   c. "The tube has a light that will allow the doctor to see your intestines."
   d. "A tube will be passed from your mouth and into your stomach."

   Rationale for your selection: ______________________________

2. The day after having a barium enema as an outpatient, the client calls the clinic nurse to express concern because the stools are white in color. Which statement made by the nurse is most helpful?
   a. "Don't worry, this is normal after a barium enema."
   b. "This is expected; be sure to drink plenty of fluids."
   c. "The stool color should return after 1 to 2 days."
   d. "This is expected; call back if your stools are still white after 5 days."

   Rationale for your selection: ______________________________

3. The nurse is taking care of a 76-year-old client who is having an upper GI series this morning. After the completion of the procedure, the nurse should initially:
   a. see whether a laxative is ordered for the client.
   b. assess the bowel sounds.
   c. take the vital signs.
   d. observe for intestinal obstruction.

   Rationale for your selection: ______________________________

ANSWER KEY FOR APPLYING CRITICAL THINKING SKILLS TO TEST QUESTIONS

HELPFUL HINTS: Read all test questions carefully. Identify key words in the question that will guide you in answering the question. In these test questions the **key words** to consider are **"correct," "most helpful,"** and **"initially."** Compare your rationale with the one in the test question.

1. The client is scheduled for a UGI endoscopy. Which statement is correct in providing the client with information about this endoscopic procedure?
   a. "A tube will be passed from your nose into your stomach."
   b. "The tube is small, is very flexible, and has a light at the end."
   c. "The tube has a light that will allow the doctor to see your intestines."
   (d.) "A tube will be passed from your mouth and into your stomach."

   Rationale: The answer is (d). This is a beginning statement that informs the client as to how the procedure will be carried out. Options (a), (b), and (c) do not provide accurate information about the procedure.

2. The day after having a barium enema as an outpatient, the client calls the clinic nurse to express concern because the stools are white in color. Which statement made by the nurse is most helpful?
   a. "Don't worry, this is normal after a barium enema."
   (b.) "This is expected; be sure to drink plenty of fluids."
   c. "The stool color should return after 1 to 2 days."
   d. "This is expected; call back if your stools are still white after 5 days."

   Rationale: The answer is (b). It is important to reassure the client and to provide instructions that help minimize complications. Barium impaction is a concern after a barium enema. Options (a), (c), and (d) do not provide enough information.

3. The nurse is taking care of a 76-year-old client who is having an upper GI series this morning. After the completion of the procedure, the nurse should initially:
   (a.) see whether a laxative is ordered for the client.
   b. assess the bowel sounds.
   c. take the vital signs.
   d. observe for intestinal obstruction.

   Rationale: The answer is (a). To prevent the complication of fecal impaction after an UGI series (barium swallow), a laxative is usually given after the procedure. Options (b) and (c) are good interventions, but the situation does not address the need for these interventions; option (d) does not focus on the initial intervention.

ONE

DIABETES MELLITUS

List the classic **signs and symptoms** of **diabetes mellitus**:

1. ______________________
2. ______________________
3. ______________________

List other **signs** and **symptoms** associated with **hyperglycemia**:

1. ______________________
2. ______________________
3. ______________________
4. ______________________
5. ______________________
6. ______________________
7. ______________________

Fill in the **circles** that identify the **signs and symptoms** associated with **hypoglycemia**.

O Polyuria O Shakiness
O Tremor
O Irritability O Glucosuria
O Polydipsia
O Sweating O Confusion
O Dizziness O Blurred vision
O Hunger
O Slurred speech
O Paresthesia O Tachycardia

Case Study: A 20-year-old woman makes an appointment with her physician for complaints of feeling fatigued and lethargic for several days. She states that she has noticed that she has lost 15 pounds. She tells the physician that she does not understand why she has lost so much weight since she has been eating a lot. The physician asks whether she voids more than usual. The client says that she does but that she thinks it is because of all the water that she is drinking all day.

Pertinent Terminology	Definition
Diabetes mellitus (DM)	
Type 1 diabetes	
Type 2 diabetes	
Insulin resistance	
Insulin	
Counterregulatory hormones	
Oral hypoglycemic agents	

The client's physician orders a fasting blood glucose (FBG) test. Another FBG and a 2-hr oral glucose tolerance test (OGTT) are also ordered. The following results are noted in the client's clinic chart. **Write** the normal laboratory value for the test in the column provided.

Test	**Results**	**Normal laboratory values**
FBG	130 mg/dL	______________________
FBG	160 mg/dL	______________________
OGTT 2-hr postload glucose	225 mg/dL	______________________

The client is informed that she has type 1 diabetes mellitus. **Fill in** the circles that correlate with the diagnosis and treatment of type 1 diabetes mellitus.

- O Oral hypoglycemics will be ordered
- O Exercise is part of the treatment plan
- O Will need to monitor for signs and symptoms of hyperglycemia
- O Insulin will be required every day
- O Will require blood glucose testing
- O Beta cells are producing insulin
- O Will need to monitor for signs and symptoms of hypoglycemia
- O Will not need insulin if follows diet

Interactive Activity: With a partner, match each question in the **follow-up case study** with the appropriate response(s) in the **Key Points Box**. Next to each question, **write** the letter(s) of the responses you have selected.

Key Points Box

A. "Usually 30 minutes to 1 hour before breakfast."
B. "Insulin needs may change over time."
C. "Check blood sugar level."
D. "Always carry oral glucose tablets."
E. "Destroyed by the gastric enzymes."
F. "No."
G. "Drink apple or grape juice."
H. "Know the signs and symptoms of hypoglycemia."

Follow-up case study: The patient is started on Humulin NPH insulin 10 units qAM and NPH 5 units qPM. She is taught how to do self-monitoring blood glucose checks (SMBG) qid.

Client's Questions	**Responses**
1. "When is the best time to administer the AM insulin?"	__________
2. "If I forget the PM dose of insulin, can I double the dose in the morning?"	__________
3. "What should I do if I begin to get shaky and dizzy?"	__________
4. "How do I prepare for a hypoglycemic reaction?"	__________

APPLYING CRITICAL THINKING SKILLS TO TEST QUESTIONS

INSTRUCTIONS: Circle the one best answer for each test question. Write your rationale for selecting the answer. To enhance your learning and test-taking skills, discuss your answer and rationale with a partner. The answer and the rationale can be found on the back of this page.

1. A client is diagnosed with diabetes mellitus type 1. In teaching the client about diabetes mellitus type 1, it is most important for the client to:
   a. know how to use hypoglycemic agents to control the diabetes.
   b. understand that insulin injections will be required daily.
   c. randomly check fingerstick blood glucose throughout the day.
   d. decrease physical activity.

   Rationale for your selection: ______________________________

2. The nurse learns in morning report that the 0700 fasting blood glucose of a client was 74 mg/dL. Which of the following morning assessment findings is of priority?
   a. Abdominal wound dressing with moderate dried red drainage.
   b. Complaining of thirst and dried mouth.
   c. Output of 250 mL during the night shift.
   d. Diaphoresis noted while taking vital signs.

   Rationale for your selection: ______________________________

3. The nurse is assigned to a client who has just been diagnosed with diabetes mellitus type 1. Which of the following assessment findings is most consistent with this diagnosis?
   a. FBG 110 mg/dL, hypertension, decreased urinary output
   b. Casual BG >140 mg/dL, obese, limited physical activity
   c. Weight loss, episodes of shakiness and diaphoresis
   d. Frequent urination, hunger, and excessive fluid intake

   Rationale for your selection: ______________________________

ANSWER KEY FOR APPLYING CRITICAL THINKING SKILLS TO TEST QUESTIONS

HELPFUL HINTS: Read all test questions carefully. Identify key words in the question that will guide you in answering the question. In these test questions the **key words** to consider are "**most important**," "**priority**," and "**most consistent.**" Compare your rationale with the one in the test question.

1. A client is diagnosed with diabetes mellitus type 1. In teaching the client about diabetes mellitus type 1, it is most important for the client to:
   a. know how to use hypoglycemic agents to control the diabetes.
   (b.) understand that insulin injections will be required daily.
   c. randomly check fingerstick blood glucose throughout the day.
   d. decrease physical activity.

   Rationale: The answer is (b). With diabetes mellitus type 1, the beta cells have stopped functioning and the use of exogenous insulin administration is required. Option (a) is not appropriate for type 1 diabetes mellitus because hypoglycemic agents are used for type 2 DM. Option (c) is incorrect because blood glucose is monitored at specific times for control; option (d) is incorrect because exercise is recommended.

2. The nurse learns in morning report that the 0700 fasting blood glucose of a client was 74 mg/dL. Which of the following morning assessment findings is of priority?
   a. Abdominal wound dressing with moderate dried red drainage.
   b. Complaining of thirst and dried mouth.
   c. Output of 250 mL during the night shift.
   (d.) Diaphoresis noted while taking vital signs.

   Rationale: The answer is (d). Diaphoresis is a sign associated with hypoglycemia and should be assessed further. Also, the morning blood glucose was toward the lower limit of normal. Options (a) and (c) are within normal limits, and option (b) is important but not a priority.

3. The nurse is assigned to a client who has just been diagnosed with diabetes mellitus type 1. Which of the following assessment findings is most consistent with this diagnosis?
   a. FBG 110 mg/dL, hypertension, decreased urinary output
   b. Casual BG > 140 mg/dL, obese, limited physical activity
   c. Weight loss, episodes of shakiness and diaphoresis
   (d.) Frequent urination, hunger, and excessive fluid intake

   Rationale: The answer is (d). The classic signs and symptoms associated with diabetes mellitus type 1 are polyuria, polydipsia, and polyphagia. Options (a), (b), and (c) are not the most consistent with the diagnosis.

COMPLICATIONS OF DIABETES MELLITUS

List the **causes** that precipitate **hypoglycemic reactions:**

1. ____________________
2. ____________________
3. ____________________
4. ____________________
5. ____________________

List the **causes** that precipitate the development of **diabetic ketoacidosis:**

1. ____________________
2. ____________________
3. ____________________

For each line identify a specific **long-term complication**, i.e., stroke, associated with diabetes mellitus.

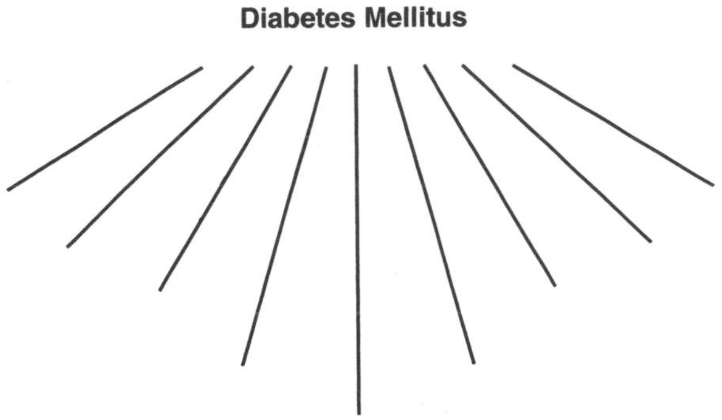

Case Study: Mr. E, 56 years old, has been a diabetic for 25 years. He is admitted to the hospital after having a cerebral vascular accident (CVA). His wife says that her husband monitors his blood glucose daily and administers his own insulin. However, she tells the nurse that he does not always stick to his diet. She wonders whether this may have contributed to the CVA. Mr. E has an order for NPH insulin 36 units qAM and NPH 17 units qPM with fingerstick blood glucose checks ac and HS. He is started on a sliding scale.

Pertinent Terminology	Definition
Lipoatrophy	
Lipohypertrophy	
Impaired glucose tolerance	
Somogyi effect	
Dawn phenomenon	
Diabetic ketoacidosis (DKA)	
Hyperglycemic hyperosmolar nonketotic coma (HHNK)	

Use the **case study, the follow-up information, and the nursing interventions below** to plan out Mr. E's morning care in the order of **priority**. Place a number, beginning with #1, in each box to indicate the sequence of the nursing care that should be delivered by the nurse.

Follow-up information: The AM blood glucose fingerstick and insulin are to be done by the morning shift. Mr. E is started on a diet containing semithick liquids.

Nursing Interventions	Rationale
☐ Perform a body systems assessment	______
☐ Perform a fingerstick blood glucose	______
☐ Take the AM vital signs	______
☐ Administer morning insulin	______
☐ Perform morning care	______
☐ Provide information regarding the complications of diabetes	______
☐ Assist with breakfast	______

Place a check (✓) next to the statements that are correct regarding the use of a sliding scale.

___ Only regular insulin is used

___ Dosage based on ac blood glucose levels

___ May be combined with other insulins

___ Used for patients with diabetes mellitus type 1

___ Used for patients with diabetes mellitus type 2

___ Used during periods of illness

Interactive Activity: The following nursing diagnosis is found on Mr. E's nursing care plan. With a partner, **write the three most important nursing interventions for the nursing diagnosis.**

Nursing Diagnosis	Nursing Interventions
Risk for aspiration r/t impaired swallowing secondary to CVA	1. ______ 2. ______ 3. ______

APPLYING CRITICAL THINKING SKILLS TO TEST QUESTIONS

INSTRUCTIONS: Circle the one best answer for each test question. Write your rationale for selecting the answer. To enhance your learning and test-taking skills, discuss your answer and rationale with a partner. The answer and the rationale can be found on the back of this page.

1. The nurse notes that the assigned client has an AV fistula on the right arm and is scheduled for hemodialysis this morning. In delegating the care of the client, it is most important for the nurse to:
   a. inform the nursing assistant to give the bath after the hemodialysis.
   b. direct that all morning care be done before hemodialysis.
   c. instruct that the blood pressure be taken on the left arm.
   d. ask that the client be weighed first.

Rationale for your selection: ______________________________

2. The nurse is admitting a client with uncontrolled diabetes mellitus. The client has left-sided hemiparesis from a previous cerebral vascular accident. The client's admitting blood glucose level was 325 mg/dL. Which of the following nursing diagnoses is of priority?
   a. Risk for fluid volume deficit
   b. Fluid volume overload
   c. Ineffective tissue perfusion
   d. Noncompliance

Rationale for your selection: ______________________________

3. The nurse is taking care of a client who has diabetes mellitus type 1. The client tells the nurse that he is beginning to feel symptoms of hypoglycemia. Which action by the nurse is of priority?
   a. Have the client drink a glass of apple juice
   b. Monitor for signs of hypoglycemia
   c. Take the pulse, respirations, and blood pressure
   d. Have the laboratory perform a blood glucose test stat

Rationale for your selection: ______________________________

ANSWER KEY FOR APPLYING CRITICAL THINKING SKILLS TO TEST QUESTIONS

HELPFUL HINTS: Read all test questions carefully. Identify key words in the question that will guide you in answering the question. In these test questions the **key words** to consider are **"most important"** and **"priority."** Compare your rationale with the one in the test question.

1. The nurse notes that the assigned client has an AV fistula on the right arm and is scheduled for hemodialysis this morning. In delegating the care of the client, it is most important for the nurse to:
   a. inform the nursing assistant to give the bath after the hemodialysis.
   b. direct that all morning care be done before hemodialysis.
   (c.) instruct that the blood pressure be taken on the left arm.
   d. ask that the client be weighed first.

Rationale: The answer is (c). It is most important to ensure the patency of the AV fistula and prevent vascular complications that can occur with applied pressure from the BP cuff. Options (a) and (b) can be done anytime, and although option (d) is important, it is not the most important on the basis of this situation.

2. The nurse is admitting a client with uncontrolled diabetes mellitus. The client has left-sided hemiparesis from a previous cerebral vascular accident. The client's admitting blood glucose level was 325 mg/dL. Which of the following nursing diagnoses is of priority?
   (a.) Risk for fluid volume deficit
   b. Fluid volume overload
   c. Ineffective tissue perfusion
   d. Noncompliance

Rationale: The answer is (a). The body will attempt to excrete the excessive glucose and will also excrete water and electrolytes, predisposing the client to dehydration. Options (b), (c), and (d) are important, but they are not priorities during the acute phase.

3. The nurse is taking care of a client who has diabetes mellitus type 1. The client tells the nurse that he is beginning to feel symptoms of hypoglycemia. Which action by the nurse is of priority?
   (a.) Have the client drink a glass of apple juice
   b. Monitor for signs of hypoglycemia
   c. Take the pulse, respirations, and blood pressure
   d. Have the laboratory perform a blood glucose test stat

Rationale: The answer is (a). The hypoglycemic effects can occur rapidly. It is always better to treat hypoglycemia in the early stages than to allow for central nervous system involvement. Options (b), (c), and (d) do not focus on the immediate treatment.

INSULIN THERAPY

List the **onset**, **peak**, and **duration** of the following insulins:

Rapid-acting:

Onset ______________________

Peak ______________________

Duration ______________________

Short-acting:

Onset ______________________

Peak ______________________

Duration ______________________

Intermediate-acting:

Onset ______________________

Peak ______________________

Duration ______________________

Long-acting:

Onset ______________________

Peak ______________________

Duration ______________________

In the boxes in the left column write (**R**) if the insulin is rapid acting, (**S**) if the insulin is short acting, (**I**) if the insulin is intermediate acting, and (**L**) if the insulin is long acting.

☐	NPH	☐
☐	Lantus (glargine)	☐
☐	NPH Iletin II	☐
☐	Humulin R	☐
☐	Humulin N	☐
☐	Humalog (lispro)	☐
☐	Novolog (aspart)	☐
☐	Apidra (glulisine)	☐
☐	Levemir (detemir)	☐

In the boxes on the right side, place an "X" to identify the insulin that may be given **IV**.

Case Study: Marty, 22 years old, has been on Humulin N insulin since her diagnosis of diabetes mellitus type 1 2 years ago. Marty administers 12 units Humulin N with 5 units Humulin R insulin qAM and 4 units Humulin N qPM. She monitors her blood glucose qid ac and HS and routinely administers the AM insulin dose at 0700 and the PM dose at 1700. Marty maintains a daily chart of her blood glucose results.

Pertinent Terminology	Definition
Glucagon	
Glycogenolysis	
Gluconeogenesis	
Glycosylated hemoglobin	
Glycosylated albumin	
Oral glucose tolerance test	
Hypoglycemia	

From the case study, plot out Marty's morning dose of Humulin N and Humulin R insulin on the **Insulin Progression Graph**. Begin with the **onset** (**O**) followed by identifying the **peak of action** (**P**) of the insulin and the **duration** (**D**).

Insulin Progression Graph
Onset → Peak → Duration

Length of time insulin remains in the body

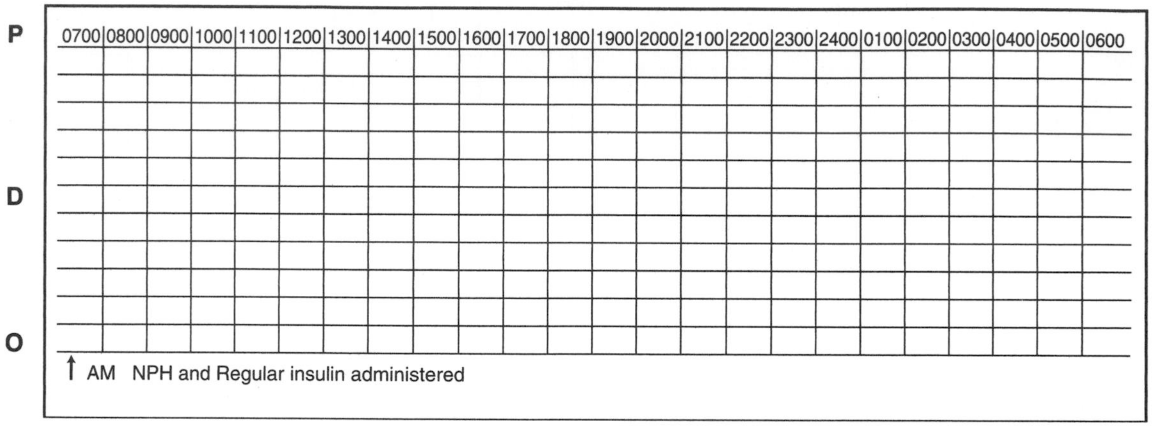

Marty eats a full breakfast 0800 but is unable to eat lunch. Use the **Insulin Progressive Graph** to indicate the time Marty would most likely experience a **hypoglycemic episode.** ________________

Select (✓) the most appropriate **snack** for Marty to eat if she experiences a hypoglycemic reaction at 1600 and has a fingerstick blood glucose of 64 mg/dl

_____ 6 saltine crackers

_____ 4 oz apple juice

_____ 8 oz diet soda

Interactive Activity: With a partner, **underline** the **correct word** in each statement as it relates to the sentence and **provide a rationale** for your selection.

1. For the patient with diabetes mellitus type 1, moderate exercise may have **hyperglycemic** or **hypoglycemic** effects.

   Rationale: ____

   ____

2. A patient with diabetes mellitus type 1 performs a fingerstick before exercising and the blood glucose results are 92 mg/dL. The patient should eat a snack **before** or **immediately after** exercising.

   Rationale: ____

   ____

   ____

3. Alcohol consumption puts the patient with diabetes mellitus type 1 at risk for **hypoglycemia** or **hyperglycemia**.

   Rationale: ____

   ____

APPLYING CRITICAL THINKING SKILLS TO TEST QUESTIONS

INSTRUCTIONS: Circle the one best answer for each test question. Write your rationale for selecting the answer. To enhance your learning and test-taking skills, discuss your answer and rationale with a partner. The answer and the rationale can be found on the back of this page.

1. The nurse learns in report that the assigned client has a fingerstick blood glucose result of 100 mg/dL at 0700. The client receives NPH insulin 15 units Sub-Q qAM. On the basis of the morning report, it is most appropriate for the nurse to:
   a. hold the AM dose of insulin.
   b. administer the AM dose of insulin.
   c. call the physician to report the blood glucose results.
   d. repeat the fingerstick blood glucose test at 0800.

   Rationale for your selection: ______________________________

2. The physician orders Humulin NPH insulin 23 units Sub-Q qAM. The nurse carries out this order correctly when the insulin:
   a. dose is given after breakfast.
   b. dose is based on the fingerstick blood glucose results.
   c. is given according to the hospital's qAM schedule.
   d. is administered before breakfast.

   Rationale for your selection: ______________________________

3. A client with diabetes mellitus type 1 had a sliding scale with regular insulin listed on the patient care rand. Based on this finding, it is most important for the nurse to:
   a. administer the regular insulin on the basis of the fasting blood glucose level.
   b. monitor the client's urine for ketones before meals.
   c. obtain fingerstick blood glucose test before meals.
   d. check the fingerstick blood glucose qid.

   Rationale for your selection: ______________________________

ANSWER KEY FOR APPLYING CRITICAL THINKING SKILLS TO TEST QUESTIONS

HELPFUL HINTS: Read all test questions carefully. Identify key words in the question that will guide you in answering the question. In these test questions the **key words** to consider are "**most appropriate,**" "**correctly,**" and "**most important.**" Compare your rationale with the one in the test question.

1. The nurse learns in report that the assigned client has a fingerstick blood glucose result of 100 mg/dL at 0700. The client receives NPH insulin 15 units Sub-Q qAM. On the basis of the morning report, it is most appropriate for the nurse to:
   a. hold the AM dose of insulin.
   (b.) administer the AM dose of insulin.
   c. call the physician to report the blood glucose results.
   d. repeat the fingerstick blood glucose test at 0800.

   Rationale: The answer is (b). The fingerstick blood glucose results are within normal limits. The nurse should administer the daily dose of insulin. Options (a), (c), and (d) are not appropriate interventions in this situation.

2. The physician orders Humulin NPH insulin 23 units Sub-Q qAM. The nurse carries out this order correctly when the insulin:
   a. dose is given after breakfast.
   b. dose is based on the fingerstick blood glucose results.
   c. is given according to the hospital's qAM schedule.
   (d.) is administered before breakfast.

   Rationale: The answer is (d). Although daily insulin is ordered qAM, the ordered dose is given before breakfast to correlate with the action of the insulin and food intake. Options (a) and (c) are similar and start after food intake. Option (b) is used mostly with regular insulin.

3. A client with diabetes mellitus type 1 had a sliding scale with regular insulin listed on the patient care rand. Based on this finding, it is most important for the nurse to:
   a. administer the regular insulin on the basis of the fasting blood glucose level.
   b. monitor the client's urine for ketones before meals.
   (c.) obtain fingerstick blood glucose test before meals.
   d. check the fingerstick blood glucose qid.

   Rationale: The answer is (c). The sliding scale is used to administer regular insulin throughout the day on the basis of fingerstick blood glucose levels. Options (a), (b), and (d) do not correlate the purpose of the sliding scale, regular insulin, blood glucose, and food intake.

LEGAL CONSIDERATIONS IN NURSING PRACTICE

List the **two types** of **torts**:

1. ______________________________
2. ______________________________

List the **four elements** that constitute **professional negligence**:

1. ______________________________
2. ______________________________
3. ______________________________
4. ______________________________

Draw a line to identify the **Unintentional Torts.**

Fraud **Invasion of privacy**

UNINTENTIONAL TORTS

Assault

Negligence

False imprisonment

Libel

Malpractice

Case Study: Cassie, a new nursing student, is assigned to Mr. W, a 73-year-old client. Mr. W has kidney disease and has been in the hospital for 3 days. He is alert and wants to know everything about his treatment and questions the nurses all the time. The change-of-shift report indicates that he has had diarrhea all day. He keeps getting out of bed, and the nurses feel that he is getting increasingly weak. Cassie is working with an experienced staff RN. The staff RN instructs Cassie to apply a vest restraint on Mr. W if he gets up again to use the bathroom because she is concerned that he will fall and injure himself.

Pertinent Terminology	Definition
Assault	
Battery	
Libel	
Slander	
Negligence	
Malpractice	
Tort	
Informed consent	
Standard of care	

Use the information in the case study to **check off** (✓) the statement or statements below that apply to the situation:

☐ A physician's order is not needed since Mr. W is increasingly weak and the nurse has determined that he is a risk to himself.

☐ A thorough neurologic assessment and documentation of unsafe behavior is important to document before applying a restraint. An order is necessary.

☐ Application of a vest restraint against Mr. W's wishes may be considered assault and battery and may have legal implications.

☐ It is important to follow the instructions of the experienced RN because she alone is responsible for the care that Mr. W receives.

Interactive Activity: With a partner, use the case studies below to (1) check off (✓) the most appropriate action(s) and (2) answer the question at the end of the case study.

Case Study

Cindi, a second-year nursing student, has been under a lot of personal stress. She tells another student that she gave her patient the wrong amount of sedative in the morning but that the patient was fine because she carefully monitored his vital signs all day. Cindi is an excellent student and will not allow this to happen again.

Action(s)

☐ The patient was fine—take no action
☐ Fill out an incident report
☐ The instructor should be notified
☐ The charge nurse should be notified

Cindi **has** or **has not** been negligent, because ______________________________
(circle one)

____

Case Study

Mark is a graduate nurse and started working as soon as he received his RN license. He administered medications one evening to a patient with a nasogastric tube. After the medication was administered, the patient began coughing and Mark noticed that the nasogastric tube was significantly out of the patient's nose.

Action(s)

☐ Notify the physician
☐ Reinsert tube and listen for placement
☐ Fill out an incident report
☐ Readminister the medications

Mark **has** or **has not** been negligent, because ______________________________
(circle one)

____

REVIEW QUESTIONS

Instructions: Select the most appropriate answer for the following multiple-choice questions.

1. The registered nurse of the medical unit is informed that four clients have dehydration and diarrhea after eating food contaminated with *E. coli*. Which nursing intervention is most effective in preventing the spread of the organism?
   a. Putting any meat found on the meal tray in the microwave for 2 minutes
   b. Wearing gloves when bathing clients and assisting the clients
   c. Assigning one nurse to care for the four clients
   d. Washing hands frequently when caring for the clients

2. A mother called the clinic nurse to ask whether her son might get head lice because he used a set of earphones 2 days ago borrowed from a friend who was just diagnosed with head lice. The nurse's instructions to the mother should include:
   a. informing her that the earphones cannot carry the head lice.
   b. having her observe her son for scratching behind the ears and back of the neck.
   c. telling her to use a lice shampoo immediately, even if head lice are not visible.
   d. informing the mother that adult head lice do not live for more than 24 hours.

3. The following vital signs are charted on the adult client's chart for the day shift: 0800, T 98, P 88 (regular), R 24, BP 128/88; 1200, T 99.4, P 92 (regular), R 22, BP 124/80. After reviewing the chart, which follow-up nursing intervention is most appropriate for the day shift nurse to implement?
   a. Retake the temperature in 1 hour.
   b. Begin cooling measures.
   c. Maintain the client on bed rest until the temperature is within the normal range.
   d. Contact the physician for an antipyretic medication.

4. The nurse is caring for a client who was admitted 2 days ago with hypertension and atrial tachycardia. The change-of-shift report indicates that the client's pulse at 0600 was 122. To apply the assessment phase of the nursing process, it is most important for the nurse to:
   a. ensure that the pulse has been reported to the physician.
   b. plan to monitor the pulse rate q2h.
   c. review the pulse rates for the last 48 hours.
   d. administer the cardiac medications on time.

5. On auscultating the lung sounds of the assigned client, the nurse hears loud vesicular breaths sounds on the anterior lateral aspects of chest during inspiration. The most appropriate follow-up action by the nurse is to:
   a. have the client use the incentive spirometer q1h while awake.
   b. monitor the client for shortness of breath q2h.
   c. check the client's pulse oximetry.
   d. document the findings.

6. The nurse auscultates the abdominal quadrants of a client and immediately hears soft gurgling bowel sounds. Which action by the nurse is most appropriate?
   a. Reassess the bowel sounds in 15 minutes.
   b. Document the findings as assessed.
   c. Chart the bowel sounds as "borborygmus."
   d. Ask another nurse to assess the bowel sounds.

7. The nurse is assigned to a client who has an indwelling urinary catheter and is placed under contact precautions. The nursing care plan indicates that the client has methicillin-resistant *Staphylococcus aureus* in the urine. To prevent the spread of infection, it is most important for the nurse to:
   a. wear a mask whenever entering the client's room.
   b. wear sterile gloves when coming in contact with the client's urine.
   c. use a gown, gloves, and mask when bathing the client.
   d. use a gown, gloves, and eye protection to empty the client's urinary catheter.

8. The nurse is bathing an elderly client at 0800. On turning the client, the nurse finds a small white tablet on the bed. The client takes Lasix (a small white tablet) at 0700 and 1700. It is most appropriate for the nurse to:
   a. document that a small white tablet was found on the client's bed.
   b. administer another dose of Lasix now.
   c. inform the client that the morning dose of Lasix was found on the bed.
   d. recommend that the medications be mixed with soft food to avoid client noncompliance.

9. An elderly client is telling the nurse the names of his grandchildren who are in a photograph. Suddenly the client begins to cry. Which action is most appropriate initially?
   a. Ask the client why he is crying.
   b. Ask the client if he would like to contact his family.
   c. Tell the client that it is difficult to be sick.
   d. Tell the client that you are sorry he feels so sad.

10. The West Nile virus is found in birds. Once the infected bird is bitten by a certain type of mosquito, the virus can then be transmitted to other birds and to humans by the mosquito. In this chain of infection, the mosquito is the:
    a. reservoir.
    b. vector.
    c. host.
    d. infectious agent.

11. The nurse writes the following expected outcome on the nursing care plan for a client who is diagnosed with a cerebral vascular accident: "The nurse will assist the client to the chair for meals every day." In applying the nursing process, this expected outcome:
    a. is written appropriately.
    b. is not measurable.
    c. should be client focused.
    d. should include how long the client may be in the chair.

12. The nurse is caring for a client who is incontinent of urine. Which nursing intervention is most effective in helping to maintain skin integrity?
    a. Change the incontinent pad q2h and prn.
    b. Limit liquid intake to 1000 mL per day.
    c. Insert an indwelling urinary catheter.
    d. Encourage daily intake of cranberry juice.

13. The nurse receives the following order for a client who is 1 day postop transurethral resection of the prostate: "Irrigate the urinary catheter with NS 0.9% until free of clots." To appropriately implement this order, the nurse would:
   a. instill 100 mL of NS 0.9% every 2 hours into the urinary catheter.
   b. manually irrigate the catheter when clots are visible in the tubing.
   c. clarify the order to include the amount of NS to use.
   d. use clean technique to irrigate the catheter.

14. The nurse is caring for an elderly client just admitted with bronchopneumonia. Which client assessment finding is of greatest concern?
   a. Respirations 26
   b. Bilateral rhonchi
   c. Acute confusion
   d. Yellow-colored sputum

15. The nursing assistant informs the registered nurse that an elderly client, recovering from a cerebral vascular accident, had some difficulty swallowing during breakfast and choked on some food. In monitoring the client for the remainder of the shift, which assessment finding requires immediate follow-up?
   a. Pulse oximetry 94
   b. 50% oral intake at noon
   c. Pulse 96 at noon; pulse 88 at 0800
   d. Temp 99.6 at noon; temp 98.6 at 0800

16. A client had a suprapubic catheter removed 2 days ago and is now being discharged. What is most important for the nurse to include in the discharge teaching?
   a. Urinary incontinence is normal for 1 to 2 weeks.
   b. Practice Kegel exercises five times per day.
   c. Empty the bladder every 2 to 3 hours for the first week.
   d. Limit fluid intake for the first week.

17. The nurse is delegating the care of a client who is 1 day postop to the nursing assistant. The nursing assistant asks whether the client's sequential stockings can be removed during the bath. Which response is most appropriate?
   a. "Do not remove the sequential stockings until tomorrow."
   b. "The sequential stockings can be removed while bathing the client."
   c. "Turn off the compression control device, but do not remove the sequential stockings."
   d. "Remove the sequential stocking as you begin to wash each leg, but reapply them immediately."

18. The nurse receives an order for bladder training for a client who has an indwelling urinary catheter. The order reads: "Clamp catheter for 2 hours, then unclamp to empty bladder, then reclamp for 2 hours." After clamping the catheter for 1 hour, the client complains of bladder discomfort and indicates a 6/10 pain level. The nurse performs a bladder scan, which shows 150 mL of urine in the bladder. Which nursing action is most appropriate initially?
   a. Unclamp the catheter and allow the bladder to empty.
   b. Review the medication record for any pain medications.
   c. Reassess the amount of urine in the bladder in 15 minutes.
   d. Inform the client of the importance of maintaining the bladder training schedule.

19. The nurse is reading the nursing care plan of a client and notices that the expected outcome was for the client to eat 90% of the regular diet by today. The change-of-shift report indicates that the client has been eating 50% of each meal for the last 24 hours. Which action by the nurse is most appropriate initially?
    a. Request the family bring in foods that the client likes.
    b. Assess the current needs of the client.
    c. Provide the client with between-meal snacks.
    d. Validate that the documentation in the chart is correct.

20. The nurse hears in report that a client has a Cheyne-Stokes breathing pattern. Which of the following would the nurse expect to see? (Select all that apply.)
    a. Periods of apnea
    b. Deep rapid breathing
    c. Shallow breathing
    d. Respiratory rate of 12 or less
    e. Full inspiration and expiration

21. The nurse is assigned to a client who receives Lasix 20 mg po BID and digoxin 0.25 mg qAM. To administer the morning dose of these drugs safely, the nurse should do which of the following? (Select all that apply.)
    a. Assess for dry mucous membranes.
    b. Expect increased serum Na^+ level.
    c. Hold the drug if diuresis noted.
    d. Monitor for decreased serum K^+ level.
    e. Take the apical pulse for 30 seconds and multiply by 2.

22. A client is 4 days postop right total hip replacement with a cemented prosthesis. To prevent right hip dislocation, it is important to tell the client which of the following? (Select all that apply.)
    a. Bend at the waist to pick up items.
    b. Do not apply any weight on the right leg.
    c. Use an elevated toilet set.
    d. Do not cross legs.
    e. Avoid lying on the right hip.

23. The nurse is caring for a client who is 3 days postop abdominal surgery. On changing the abdominal dressing, the nurse notes the surgical incision has eviscerated. The nurse is correct in doing which of the following? (Select all that apply.)
    a. Keep the client on bed rest.
    b. Apply a dry sterile dressing on the wound.
    c. Monitor vital signs q2h.
    d. Place a moist dressing on the wound.
    e. Encourage fluid intake.

24. The nurse is assigned to care for a client diagnosed with diabetes mellitus type 1. The physician orders Lantus insulin 22 units qPM, fingerstick blood glucose testing ac and HS, and a sliding scale with Regular insulin. To appropriately implement the sliding scale order, when will the nurse administer Regular insulin? (Select all that apply.)
    a. Every time the fingerstick blood glucose is tested
    b. On the basis of the fingerstick blood glucose results
    c. 30 minutes after each meal and at the hour of sleep
    d. In combination with the Lantus insulin PM dose
    e. 5 units before each meal and at the hour of sleep

25. The nurse admits an adult client diagnosed with a bowel obstruction. The physician writes the following orders: (1) NPO, (2) insert a nasogastric tube to low wall suction. To implement the orders, the nurse would do which of the following? (Select all that apply.)
    a. Use a 10 Fr nasogastric tube
    b. Use a 14 Fr nasogastric tube
    c. Provide the client with water during insertion of the nasogastric tube
    d. Manually aspirate all gastric contents immediately after nasogastric tube insertion
    e. Ensure that the nasogastric tube is connected to the suction equipment before inserting the tube

Section Two - Priority-Setting and Decision-Making Activities

STANDARDS OF PROFESSIONAL PERFORMANCE

Identify the Standards of Professional Performance

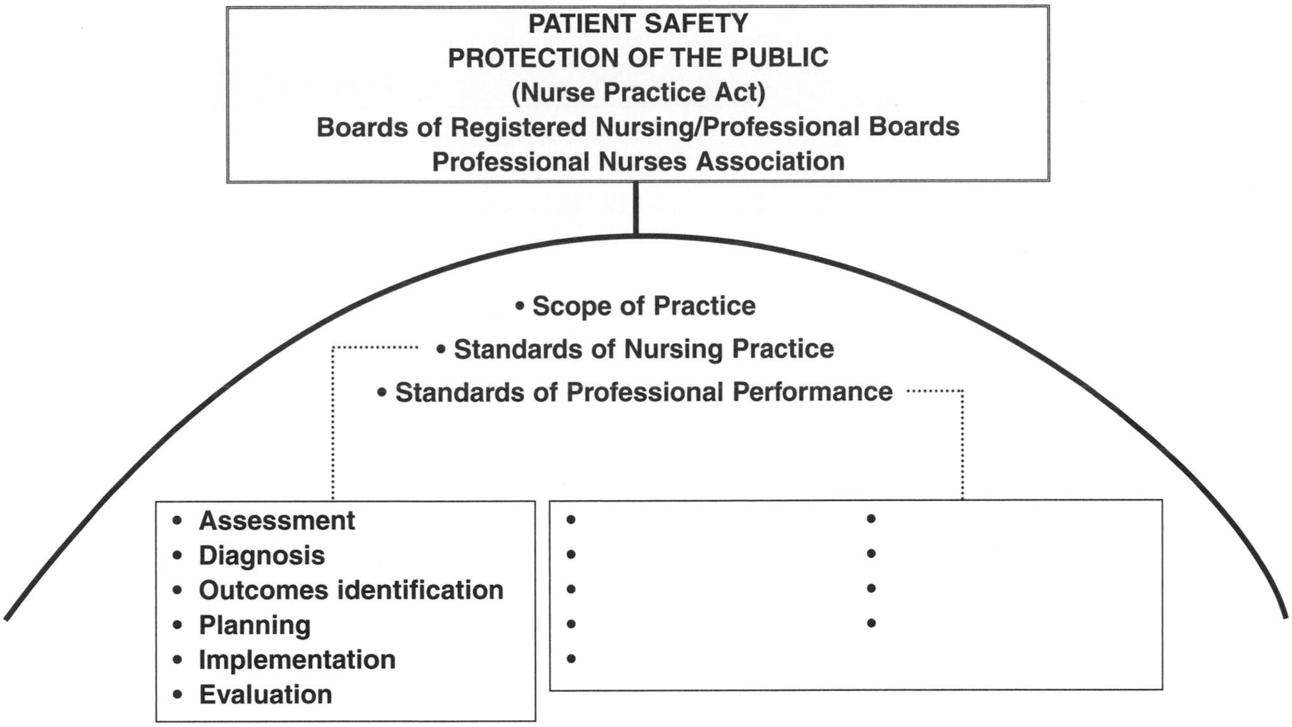

Case Study: The RN on the medical-surgical unit has been a staff member for 15 years. She is clinically very competent and establishes good rapport with clients and their families. The RN has currently been assigned to work with nursing students. Several of the students have complained that it is difficult to work with this RN because she prefers to work independently and rarely answers the student's questions. The RN has commented to other staff that she only agreed to take students because the supervisor wants nursing students on the unit.

Pertinent Terminology	Definition
American Nurses Association (ANA)	______________________
Canadian Nurses Association (CNA)	______________________
Standards of nursing practice	______________________
Standards of professional performance	______________________

- Use the ANA Standards of Professional Performance to identify the behaviors that represent professional performance.
- Use the case study to put an "X" in the middle column, which identifies the staff RN's professional performance behaviors that needs strengthening.

ANA Standards of Professional Performance		**Write in behaviors that describe professional performance for each standard.**
Quality of Practice		
Education		
Practice Evaluation		
Collegiality		
Collaboration		
Ethics		
Research		
Resource Utilization		
Leadership		

Interactive Activity: With a partner, discuss the following statements related to "standards." **Underline** the statements that are **TRUE.**

1. Standards, such as the Standards of Nursing Practice and Standards of Professional Practice, are considered legally binding regulations.

2. Standards of Nursing Practice can be used in a court of law in malpractice cases.

3. Standards of Nursing Practice identify the minimal expectations in the delivery of nursing care.

4. Professional nurses working in the outpatient setting are not held to the same standards of nursing practice as are professional nurses working in the acute care setting.

5. Additional standards of nursing care may be required in specialty areas such as medical-surgical units, pediatric units, and critical care units.

THE PATIENT UNDERGOING SURGERY

Mr. H, age 60 years, was admitted with persistent abdominal pain. He states he has had nausea and vomiting and has noticed a 10-pound weight loss within the last 2 months. He is diagnosed with gastric cancer and is scheduled for a subtotal gastrectomy in the morning. He has morphine sulfate 10 mg q3h IV prn, promethazine 25 mg IV q4hr prn nausea, and Mylanta 30 mL po q2h prn abdominal pain. Mr. H is very anxious after speaking with his physician and refuses to sign the surgical consent. He tells the nurse that he is having abdominal pain and "wants his pain shot right now." The nurse notes that it is just about 3 hours since his last pain medication and the Mylanta was given 2 hours ago.

Instructions: Prioritize the following **nursing interventions** as you, the nurse, would do them to initially take care of Mr. H. Write a number in the box to identify the order of your interventions (#1 = first intervention, #2 = second intervention, etc.) and state a **rationale** for each intervention.

INTERVENTIONS	PRIORITY #	RATIONALE
• Administer IV pain med.	☐	______
• Sit and talk with patient	☐	______
• Give Mylanta 30 mL	☐	______
• Offer to call a family member	☐	______
• Notify physician	☐	______

KEY POINTS TO CONSIDER: ______

Mr. H does consent to have surgery and returns to the medical unit postoperatively. He has an IV of lactated Ringer's solution infusing at 125 mL/hr, and you note the following:

1. P 90, R 20, BP 130/76
2. He is alert and oriented and his skin is warm and dry
3. NG tube draining brown-reddish drainage (300 mL in the last 4 hours)
4. Indwelling urinary catheter draining light yellow urine (700 mL in the last 4 hours)

Interactive activity: With a partner, **do the following: (1) on the basis of the current assessment, select** the **one nursing diagnosis** that is of priority at this time, **(2) provide a rationale** for your selection, and **(3) list three nursing interventions** that meet the needs of Mr. H:

All of the following nursing diagnoses may apply to Mr. H:

Risk for infection, Pain, Anxiety, Ineffective airway clearance, Fatigue, Impaired physical mobility, Imbalanced nutrition: less than body requirements, Deficient knowledge, Risk for deficient fluid volume, Fear

Nursing Diagnosis	Rationale	Nursing Interventions

Several hours after surgery you note that Mr. H is very restless and you assess: R 32, P 130, BP 108/70, NG drainage 200 mL bright red drainage, skin cool, c/o pain

Instructions: Based on the situation, identify and write the **priority problem** in the box below. Then, starting with the small box labeled **#1, prioritize** the **nursing interventions** for this situation and identify your plan for follow-up care for Mr. H.

NURSING INTERVENTIONS

A. Monitor P, R, BP, and pulse oximetry

B. Document assessment/nursing care

C. Prepare for gastric lavage

D. Plan to start oxygen therapy

E. Stay with Mr. H

F. Notify physician

DECISION-MAKING DIAGRAM

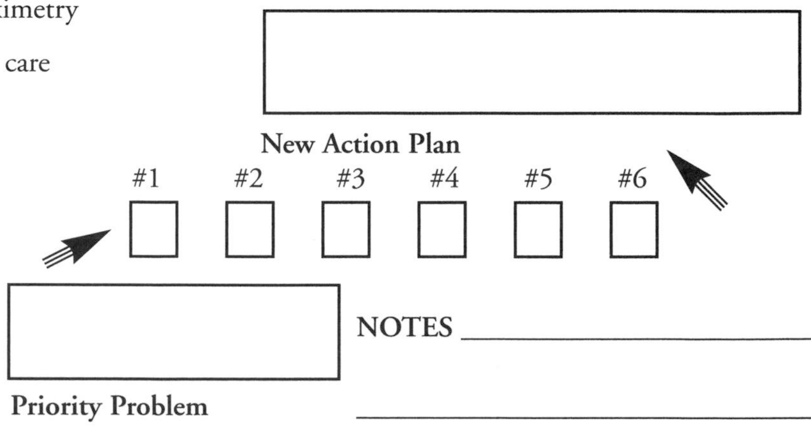

NOTES ______________________

____

APPLYING CRITICAL THINKING SKILLS TO TEST QUESTIONS

INSTRUCTIONS: Circle the one best answer for each test question. Write your rationale for selecting the answer. To enhance your learning and test-taking skills, discuss your answer and rationale with a partner. The answer and the rationale can be found on the back of this page.

TWO

1. The nurse assesses the following on a client who had a colon resection 5 days ago: I & O × 4, skin warm, abd distended nontender, bowel sounds present. Abd sutures approximated. States pain level 2. IV infusing at 75 mL/hr per pump. Fine crackles in the bilateral lower lung bases. In planning care, which nursing action is of priority?
   a. Take vital signs q4h
   b. Ambulate the client
   c. Assess lung sounds q4h
   d. Push oral fluids

   Rationale: ____________________

2. The nurse is caring for a client who has diabetes mellitus type 1 and is 2 days postop abdominal surgery. The client takes clopidrogrel (Plavix) 75 mg po daily and aspirin 81 mg po daily. In preparing the administration of these drugs, it is most important for the nurse to first:
   a. assess whether the client is having mild pain.
   b. check the serum prothrombin time levels.
   c. monitor the blood pressure.
   d. ensure that the client has eaten.

   Rationale: ____________________

3. The nurse administers atropine 0.4 mg IM as ordered preop for surgery. Thirty minutes after administration, the client complains of a very dry mouth and has flushed, dry skin with an oral temperature of 99° F and a pulse rate of 104. The most appropriate nursing action is for the nurse to:
   a. document the client's complaints.
   b. notify the physician.
   c. take the client's temperature in 1 hour.
   d. recognize that these are normal side effects of the drug.

   Rationale: ____________________

ANSWER KEY FOR APPLYING CRITICAL THINKING SKILLS TO TEST QUESTIONS

HELPFUL HINTS: Read all test questions carefully. Identify key words in the question that will guide you in answering the question. In these test questions the **key words** to consider are "**priority,**" "**most important,**" and "**most appropriate.**" Compare your rationale with the one in the test question.

1. The nurse assesses the following on a client who had a colon resection 5 days ago: I & O × 4, skin warm, abd distended nontender, bowel sounds present. Abd sutures approximated. States pain level 2. IV infusing at 75 mL/hr per pump. Fine crackles in the bilateral lower lung bases. In planning care, which nursing action is of priority?
   a. Take vital signs q4h
   (b.) Ambulate the client
   c. Assess lung sounds q4h
   d. Push oral fluids

   Rationale: The answer is (b). Assessment data indicate the need to ambulate the client to ease abdominal distention and enhance respiration and movement of secretions. Options (a), (c), and (d) are important but do not help the client with the priority problems.

2. The nurse is caring for a client who has diabetes mellitus type 1 and is 2 days postop abdominal surgery. The client takes clopidrogrel (Plavix) 75 mg po daily and aspirin 81 mg po daily. In preparing the administration of these drugs, it is most important for the nurse to first:
   a. assess whether the client is having mild pain.
   (b.) check the serum prothrombin time levels.
   c. monitor the blood pressure.
   d. ensure that the client has eaten.

   Rationale: The answer is (b). Clopidrogrel and aspirin both have anticoagulation properties. Coagulation studies should be monitored throughout therapy. Options (a), (c), and (d) do not address the most important intervention related to this drug therapy.

3. The nurse administers atropine 0.4 mg IM as ordered preop for surgery. Thirty minutes after administration, the client complains of a very dry mouth and has flushed, dry skin with an oral temperature of 99° F and a pulse rate of 104. The most appropriate nursing action is for the nurse to:
   a. document the client's complaints.
   (b.) notify the physician.
   c. take the client's temperature in 1 hour.
   d. recognize that these are normal side effects of the drug.

   Rationale: The answer is (b). Atropine is a cholinergic blocking agent. The client is manifesting symptoms of adverse effects. Options (a) and (c) are not the most important.There is a narrow margin between the side effects and the adverse effects of the drug. The nurse should research the drug literature before selecting option (d).

THE PATIENT WITH AN INTESTINAL OBSTRUCTION

Mrs. W, 56 years old, is hospitalized with the diagnosis of small bowel obstruction. She has an NG tube to low continuous suction draining dark brown drainage and an IV of D5/0.45 NS with 30 mEq potassium chloride (Kcl) infusing at 100 mL/hr. Her skin is warm and dry and her mucous membranes are dry. Her abdomen is distended with hyperactive bowel sounds in the right upper and lower quadrants. The nursing assistant reports that Mrs. W. just vomited 100 mL of dark brown secretions.

Instructions: Prioritize the following **nursing interventions** as you would do them to initially take care of Mrs. W. Write a number in the box to identify the order of your interventions (#1 = first intervention, #2 = second intervention, etc.) and state a **rationale** for each intervention.

INTERVENTIONS	PRIORITY #	RATIONALE
• Provide thorough mouth care	☐	______
• Assess abdomen, measure abdominal girth	☐	______
• Assess NG tube and suction	☐	______
• Take the vital signs	☐	______
• Ensure Mrs. W is in semi-Fowler's position	☐	______

KEY POINTS TO CONSIDER: ______

After 48 hours Mrs. W's abdomen is less distended and the current assessment findings include:

1. Hemoglobin 9.2 g, hematocrit 29%, K^+ 3.1 mEq , Na^+ 145 mEq
2. T 98.8° F, P 92, irregular, R 20, BP 152/94
3. NG tube draining dark brown drainage (250 mL in the last 8 hours)
4. Pain on a 0-10 scale = 4
5. No stool or passing of flatus, urine output last 24 hr 700 mL

Interactive activity: With a partner, **do the following:** (1) **based on the current assessment, select** the **one nursing diagnosis** that is of priority at this time, (2) **provide a rationale** for your selection, and (3) **list three nursing interventions** that meet the needs of Mrs. W.

All the following nursing diagnoses may apply to Mrs. W:

Risk for infection, Pain, Anxiety, Ineffective airway clearance, Imbalanced nutrition: less than body requirements, Deficient knowledge, Deficient fluid volume, Risk for impaired skin integrity, Fear, Disturbed sleep pattern

Nursing Diagnosis	Rationale	Nursing Interventions

The next day, Mrs. W's assessment included the following: NG output 500 mL and urine output 100 mL dark amber during the night shift. Faint bowel sounds, capillary refill >5 seconds. Weak, lethargic, and disoriented. Mucous membranes dry. Orthostatic BP 148/90 (lying) 124/84 (standing).

Instructions: On the basis of the situation, identify and write the **priority problem** in the box below. Then, starting with the small box labeled #1, **prioritize** the **nursing interventions** for this situation and identify your follow-up action plan for Mrs. W.

NURSING INTERVENTIONS

A. Monitor IV fluid replacement

B. Inform physician

C. Orient Mrs. W

D. Provide oral care

E. Raise side rails

F. Take vital signs

DECISION-MAKING DIAGRAM

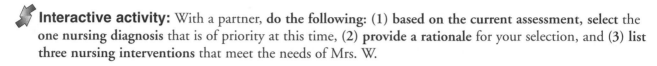

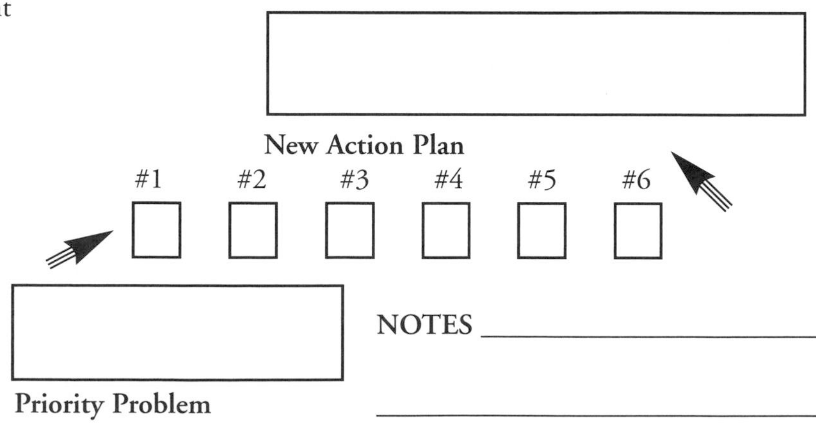

NOTES ____________________

____

APPLYING CRITICAL THINKING SKILLS TO TEST QUESTIONS

INSTRUCTIONS: **Circle the one best answer for each test question.** Write your rationale for selecting the answer. To enhance your learning and test-taking skills, discuss your answer and rationale with a partner. The answer and the rationale can be found on the back of this page.

1. The nurse is taking care of a client who has an NG tube to continuous low suction. The nursing assistant reports that the client has vomited 100 mL of light yellow-greenish fluid. It is most important for the nurse to initially:
   a. check the medication record for an antiemetic.
   b. check the NG tube placement.
   c. add the emesis to the total output for the shift.
   d. ask the client whether the desire to vomit has stopped.

   Rationale: ______________________________

2. The nurse is caring for a client who was admitted with upper gastrointestinal bleeding. The client has an NG tube to continuous low suction and has an order for Mylanta 30 mL by NG tube q4h. The nurse administers 30 mL of Mylanta at 0900. A priority follow-up nursing intervention is to
   a. maintain the tube to low continuous suction.
   b. document medication administration.
   c. ensure NG tube placement.
   d. clamp the NG tube for 30 minutes.

   Rationale: ______________________________

3. The client is receiving continuous full-strength formula tube feeding through an NG feeding tube at 75 mL/hr, and there is 100 mL left in the feeding bag. The nurse is preparing to administer the 0900 routine medications through the feeding tube. Which technique is best for administering the 0900 medications?
   a. Crush the medications, dissolve in water, and put in the feeding bag.
   b. Crush the medications, dissolve in water, and give using a 50-mL syringe.
   c. Crush the medications, dissolve in water, and check tube placement.
   d. Crush the medications, dissolve in water, and check residual before giving.

   Rationale: ______________________________

TWO

ANSWER KEY FOR APPLYING CRITICAL THINKING SKILLS TO TEST QUESTIONS

HELPFUL HINTS: Read all test questions carefully. Identify key words in the question that will guide you in answering the question. In these test questions the **key words** to consider are **"most important," "priority,"** and **"best."** Compare your rationale with the one found for each question.

1. The nurse is taking care of a client who has an NG tube to continuous low suction. The nursing assistant reports that the client has vomited 100 mL of light yellow-greenish fluid. It is most important for the nurse to initially:
   a. check the medication record for an antiemetic.
   (b.) check the NG tube placement.
   c. add the emesis to the total output for the shift.
   d. ask the client whether the desire to vomit has stopped.

   Rationale: The answer is (b). Vomiting should not be experienced with the use of an NG tube. Tube placement should be assessed. Option (a) is not the initial intervention and options (c) and (d) are not the most important interventions.

2. The nurse is caring for a client who was admitted with upper gastrointestinal bleeding. The client has an NG tube to continuous low suction and has an order for Mylanta 30 mL by NG tube q4h. The nurse administers 30 mL of Mylanta at 0900. A priority follow-up nursing intervention is to
   a. maintain the tube to low continuous suction.
   b. document medication administration.
   c. ensure NG tube placement.
   (d.) clamp the NG tube for 30 minutes.

   Rationale: The answer is (d). It is important to clamp the tube for 30 minutes to allow for drug absorption. Option (a) is an ongoing nursing action, option (b) should be done after drug administration, and option (c) should have been done before drug administration.

3. The client is receiving continuous full-strength formula tube feeding through an NG feeding tube at 75 mL/hr, and there is 100 mL left in the feeding bag. The nurse is preparing to administer the 0900 routine medications through the feeding tube. Which technique is best in administering the 0900 medications?
   a. Crush the medications, dissolve in water, and put in the feeding bag.
   b. Crush the medications, dissolve in water, and give using a 50-mL syringe.
   (c.) Crush the medications, dissolve in water, and check tube placement.
   d. Crush the medications, dissolve in water, and check residual before giving.

   Rationale: The answer is (c). Tube placement should be checked before administration of medication or formula feeding. Options (a), (b), and (d) do not describe the best technique.

THE PATIENT WITH A COLOSTOMY

Mrs. P, 42 years old, had surgery today for colon cancer. She was transferred to her room 2 hours ago. In the evening shift report you learn that she had a sigmoid colostomy and has a colostomy bag in place, a clean dry surgical dressing, an NG tube to low continuous wall suction draining dark brown drainage, a right central line with total parenteral nutrition (TPN) infusing at 83 mL/hr, and an IV of D5/NS with a PCA (morphine sulfate) set to deliver 1 mg/6 min per patient demand.

Instructions: Prioritize the following **nursing interventions** as you, the nurse, would do them to initially take care of Mrs. P. Write a number in the box to identify the order of your interventions (#1 = first intervention, #2 = second intervention, etc.) and state a **rationale** for each intervention.

INTERVENTIONS	PRIORITY #	RATIONALE
• Assess surgical dressing and stoma	☐	______________________
• Take the vital signs	☐	______________________
• Assess pain level	☐	______________________
• Check NG tube and drainage	☐	______________________
• Check IV site, TPN and PCA setting	☐	______________________

KEY POINTS TO CONSIDER: ______________________

____

____

The **first postop day** assessment was significant for the following signs and symptoms:

1. Bowel sounds absent
2. Mrs. P moans when she turns in bed
3. Weak, ineffective cough
4. Stoma swollen and reddened

Interactive activity: With a partner, **do the following:** (1) **select** the **one nursing diagnosis** that is of priority at this time, (2) **provide a rationale** for your selection, and (3) **list three nursing interventions** that assist to meet the needs of the patient:

All of the following nursing diagnoses may apply to Mrs. P:

> Risk for infection, Risk for impaired skin integrity, Pain, Anxiety, Ineffective airway clearance, Fatigue, Impaired physical mobility, Imbalanced nutrition: less than body requirements, Disturbed body image, Risk for deficient fluid volume, Fear

Nursing Diagnosis	Rationale	Nursing Interventions

On the morning of the **third postop day**, the NG tube was removed per the physician's orders and Mrs. P was started on a clear liquid diet. In the afternoon the assessment findings included: Stoma edematous and pale, abdomen distended, complaints of pain.

Instructions: On the basis of the **third postop day** assessment, identify and write the **priority problem** in the box below. Then, starting with the small box labeled **#1, prioritize** the **nursing interventions** listed and **identify** your action plan for the follow-up care of Mrs. P.

NURSING INTERVENTIONS

A. Take the vital signs

B. Prepare to insert NG tube

C. Assess colostomy bag and bowel sounds

D. Notify physician stat

E. Place on NPO

F. Check IV patency

DECISION-MAKING DIAGRAM

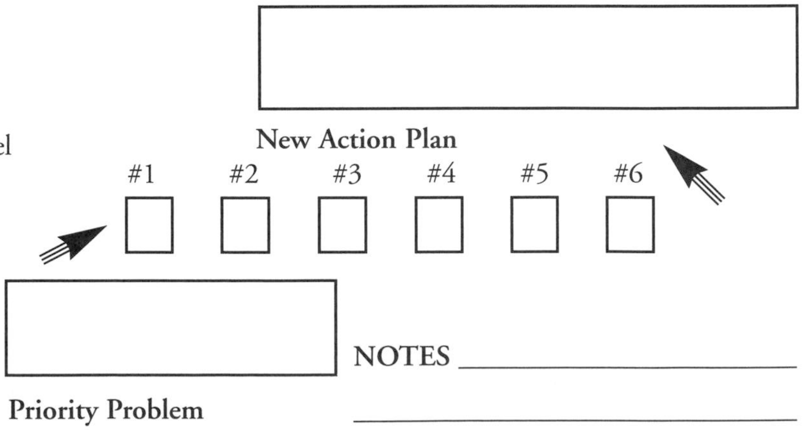

APPLYING CRITICAL THINKING SKILLS TO TEST QUESTIONS

INSTRUCTIONS: Circle the one best answer for each test question. Write your rationale for selecting the answer. To enhance your learning and test-taking skills, discuss your answer and rationale with a partner. The answer and the rationale can be found on the back of this page.

TWO

1. The patient care rand (Kardex) of a client indicates that a double-barrel colostomy was performed 2 days ago. Which assessment finding is of most concern?
   a. Right-sided colostomy bag with small amount fecal drainage, left-sided colostomy bag with serosanguineous mucous drainage.
   b. Right-sided colostomy bag with serosanguineous mucous drainage. Stoma dark red. Left-sided colostomy bag with minimal drainage.
   c. Abdomen soft, tender to touch, stomas red and edematous.
   d. Bowel sounds hypoactive on right side; absent on left side.

   Rationale: ______________________________

2. The nurse is assigned to a client who was had an ileostomy 3 days ago and now has rales in the upper lung fields. The client is receiving IV fluid set at 75 mL/hr. Which of the following interventions is most important for the nurse to ask the nursing assistant to perform?
   a. Take vital signs q4h
   b. Monitor intake and output q8h
   c. Push 500 mL of fluid for the shift
   d. Assist the client to turn in bed q4h

   Rationale: ______________________________

3. The client is 72 years old and is admitted with a respiratory tract infection. The client is on erythromycin 400 mg q6h po. The client has a sigmoid colostomy. Which of the following assessment findings would be most indicative of a potential complication?
   a. Admission white blood count of 11,500
   b. Six liquid stools during the shift
   c. T 100.8° F during morning assessment
   d. Urinary output of 260 mL for the last 4 hours

   Rationale: ______________________________

ANSWER KEY FOR APPLYING CRITICAL THINKING SKILLS TO TEST QUESTIONS

HELPFUL HINTS: Read all test questions carefully. Identify key words in the question that will guide you in answering the question. In these test questions the **key words** to consider are **"most concern," "most important,"** and **"most indicative."** Compare your rationale with the one found for each question.

1. The patient care rand (Kardex) of a client indicates that a double-barrel colostomy was performed 2 days ago. Which assessment finding is of most concern?
   a. Right-sided colostomy bag with small amount fecal drainage, left-sided colostomy bag with serosanguineous mucous drainage.
   (b.) Right-sided colostomy bag with serosanguineous mucous drainage. Stoma dark red. Left-sided colostomy bag with minimal drainage.
   c. Abdomen soft, tender to touch, stomas red and edematous.
   d. Bowel sounds hypoactive on right side; absent on left side.

   Rationale: The answer is (b). The dark red color of the stoma is an indication of possible impaired perfusion of the stoma. Options (a), (c), and (d) are normal assessment findings consistent with the situation.

2. The nurse is assigned to a client who was had an ileostomy 3 days ago and now has rales in the upper lung fields. The client is receiving IV fluid set at 75 mL/hr. Which of the following interventions is most important for the nurse to ask the nursing assistant to perform?
   a. Take vital signs q4h
   b. Monitor intake and output q8h
   (c.) Push 500 mL of fluid for the shift
   d. Assist the client to turn in bed q4h

   Rationale: The answer is (c). A new ileostomy will initially drain up to 2 L/day. Replacing fluid to prevent dehydration is important. Options (a), (b), and (d) are good interventions, but the client needs hydration because of the fluid loss.

3. The client is 72 years old and is admitted with a respiratory tract infection. The client is on erythromycin 400 mg q6h po. The client has a sigmoid colostomy. Which of the following assessment findings would be most indicative of a potential complication?
   a. Admission white blood count of 11,500
   (b.) Six liquid stools during the shift
   c. T 100.8° F during morning assessment
   d. Urinary output of 260 mL for the last 4 hours

   Rationale: The answer is (b). Erythromycin can cause diarrhea. With a sigmoid colostomy the client should have near-to-normal stools. Options (a) and (c) are symptoms associated with an infection, for which the client was admitted. Option (d) is within normal limits.

THE PATIENT WITH COLON CANCER

Mr. S, 65 years old, has colon cancer. He is admitted for a colon resection. His current medical history is significant for complaints of changes in bowel habits/constipation, passing of bloody stools, abdominal pain, and weight loss. His past medical condition includes a history of coronary artery disease and hypertension. In addition to antihypertensive medication, he takes aspirin 81 mg po daily. In preparation for surgery, his current orders include NPO, insert an NG tube, and a saline lock. His 6:00 AM vital signs are T 98° F, P 78, R 20, BP 162/90. He is to receive his preop medication at 12:00 noon today. The nurse completes report at 8:00 AM.

Instructions: Prioritize the five **nursing interventions** as you, the nurse, would do them to initially take care of Mr. S. Write a number in the box to identify the order of your interventions (#1 = first intervention, #2 = second intervention, etc.) and state a **rationale** for each intervention.

INTERVENTIONS	PRIORITY #	RATIONALE
• Perform a body systems assessment	☐	______
• Take the vital signs	☐	______
• Insert saline lock	☐	______
• Insert NG tube	☐	______
• Check surgical consent	☐	______

KEY POINTS TO CONSIDER: ______

______

______

TWO

A colon resection is done on Mr. S. The **first postop day** assessment includes:

1. Lactated Ringer's infusing at 100 mL/hr and PCA with morphine sulfate
2. Elastic stockings on; intermittent compression device ordered for 24 hours
3. NG tube to low continuous wall suction draining brown-greenish fluid
4. Wants to stay in a low-Fowler's position
5. Short and shallow respirations

Interactive activity: With a partner, **do the following:** (1) based on the **first postop day assessment, select** the **one nursing diagnosis** that is a priority at this time, (2) **provide a rationale** for your selection, and (3) **list three nursing interventions** that meet the needs of Mr. S.

All of the following nursing diagnoses may apply to Mr. S:

Risk for infection, Pain, Anxiety, Ineffective airway clearance, Imbalanced nutrition: less than body requirements, Deficient knowledge, Risk for deficient fluid volume, Risk for impaired skin integrity, Risk for ineffective tissue perfusion, Fear

Nursing Diagnosis	Rationale	Nursing Interventions

On the **fourth postoperative day** you assess the following signs and symptoms on Mr. S: Complaints of tenderness in the right calf with a positive Homan's sign, 2+ right ankle/calf edema, right calf is warmer to touch than the left calf.

Instructions: Based on the **fourth postoperative day** assessment, identify and write the **priority problem** in the box below. Then, starting with the small box labeled #1, **prioritize** the **nursing interventions** listed and **identify** your action plan for the follow-up care of Mr. S.

NURSING INTERVENTIONS

- **A.** Elevate right extremity
- **B.** Notify physician
- **C.** Maintain bed rest
- **D.** Allay Mr. S's concerns
- **E.** Administer mild analgesic if ordered
- **F.** Assess pedal pulses

DECISION-MAKING DIAGRAM

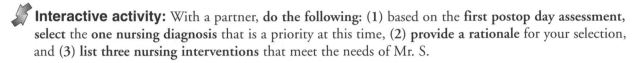

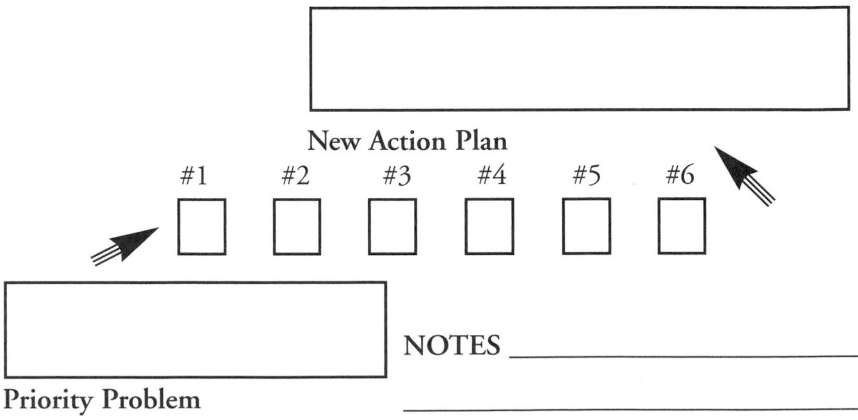

NOTES

APPLYING CRITICAL THINKING SKILLS TO TEST QUESTIONS

INSTRUCTIONS: Circle the one best answer for each test question. Write your rationale for selecting the answer. To enhance your learning and test-taking skills, discuss your answer and rationale with a partner. The answer and the rationale can be found on the back of this page.

1. The nurse is caring for a client who had a ileostomy 5 days ago. The ileostomy is draining large amounts of green-brownish liquid stool. On discharge, the client asks the nurse whether the stool consistency will eventually become more solid. Which response by the nurse is best?
   a. "The stool will become solid as the ileostomy heals."
   b. "Eating certain foods can help make the stool more solid."
   c. "It takes about 1 year to see exactly what the stool consistency will be."
   d. "The stool will change to a mushy consistency after several months."

   Rationale: ____

2. The nurse is providing discharge instructions to a client who is going home after having an ileostomy for colon cancer. A priority discharge instruction is to instruct the client to
   a. irrigate the ileostomy weekly.
   b. drink eight glasses of water daily.
   c. monitor the daily output from the ileostomy.
   d. use a mild laxative if there is no ileostomy drainage for 24 hours.

   Rationale: ____

3. The nurse is assisting a client to irrigate his colostomy. After instilling the water, the client has no output. What should the nurse do next?
   a. Encourage the client to ambulate
   b. Irrigate the colostomy again within 30 minutes
   c. Digitally stimulate the colostomy opening
   d. Notify the physician

   Rationale: ____

ANSWER KEY FOR APPLYING CRITICAL THINKING SKILLS TO TEST QUESTIONS

HELPFUL HINTS: Read all test questions carefully. Identify key words in the question that will guide you in answering the question. In these test questions the **key words** to consider are **"best," "priority,"** and **"next."** Compare your rationale with the one in the test question.

1. The nurse is caring for a client who had a ileostomy 5 days ago. The ileostomy is draining large amounts of green-brownish liquid stool. On discharge, the client asks the nurse whether the stool consistency will eventually become more solid. Which response by the nurse is best?
   a. "The stool will become solid as the ileostomy heals."
   b. "Eating certain foods can help make the stool more solid."
   c. "It takes about 1 year to see exactly what the stool consistency will be."
   (d.) "The stool will change to a mushy consistency after several months."

   Rationale: The answer is (d). Fecal drainage from an ileostomy is mostly liquid and changes to a mushy consistency in 3 to 6 months. Options (a), (b), and (c) do not provide the client with the correct information.

2. The nurse is providing discharge instructions to a client who is going home after having an ileostomy for colon cancer. A priority discharge instruction is to instruct the client to
   a. irrigate the ileostomy weekly.
   (b.) drink eight glasses of water daily.
   c. monitor the daily output from the ileostomy.
   d. use a mild laxative if there is no ileostomy drainage for 24 hours.

   Rationale: The answer is (b). Daily fecal drainage from a new ileostomy can range from 1000 to 2000 mL. The client is at risk for dehydration along with fluid and electrolyte imbalance. Options (a) and (d) are interventions that do not apply to the care of an ileostomy. Option (c) is good but does not help the client prevent a complication.

3. The nurse is assisting a client to irrigate his colostomy. After instilling the water, the client has no output. What should the nurse do next?
   (a.) Encourage the client to ambulate
   b. Irrigate the colostomy again within 30 minutes
   c. Digitally stimulate the colostomy opening
   d. Notify the physician

   Rationale: The answer is (a). Ambulation can stimulate peristalsis and the flow of fecal drainage. Option (b) would instill more fluid and may cause trauma and excessive loss of fluid and electrolytes. Option (c) is not appropriate, and option (d) is not necessary because it may take some time for the drainage to begin.

THE PATIENT WITH TOTAL PARENTERAL NUTRITION

You are assigned to care for Mrs. F. In report you learn that her diarrhea is decreasing and her current vital signs (VS) are T 98.8° F, P 76, R 18, BP 130/84. She has complained of pain in her right leg.

VS q4h I & O (✓) Weigh qAM BRP with assist prn Admit date: 3/16 Name: F, J. M. Age: 55	Right central line inserted 3/16 TPN @ 83 mL/hr per IV pump Lipids 10% (M-W-F) BG Fingersticks q6h (6-12-6-12) Dx: Dehydration/Diarrhea Hx of Crohn's—acute exacerbation, atrial fibrillation	Diet: NPO Routine med: Vit. K 10 mg Sub-Q qMon Regular Insulin 2 units if BG = 180 – 200 mg Call MD if BG more than 200 mg

Instructions: Prioritize the five **nursing interventions** as you would do them to take care of Mrs. F. Write a number in the box to identify the order of your interventions (#1 = first intervention, #2 = second intervention, etc.) and state a **rationale** for each intervention.

INTERVENTIONS	PRIORITY #	RATIONALE
• Perform a body systems physical assessment	☐	______
• Assess right leg	☐	______
• Assess central line for patency and central line dressing	☐	______
• Get 0600 blood glucose results	☐	______
• Assess right arm and neck for distention	☐	______

KEY POINTS TO CONSIDER: ______

Mrs. F was taken to x-ray 1 hour ago. On her return to the unit, the IV pump is beeping and you are informed that the machine has been beeping for a long time. You assess the following:

1. TPN not infusing
2. Skin warm, diaphoretic, complaints of nervousness and rapid heartbeat
3. VS: T 98° F, P 118, R 26, BP 136/80

 Interactive activity: With a partner, **do the following: (1) select** the **one nursing diagnosis** that is of priority at this time, **(2) provide a rationale** for your selection, and **(3) list the nursing interventions** that assist to meet the needs of the patient:

All of the following nursing diagnoses may apply to Mrs. F:

> Anxiety, Risk for infection, Risk for activity intolerance, Risk for excess fluid volume, Impaired tissue integrity, Ineffective tissue perfusion, Imbalanced nutrition: less than body requirements, Risk for injury: hypoglycemia, Deficient knowledge

Nursing Diagnosis	Rationale	Nursing Interventions

Three hours later, Mrs. F's family comes to the nursing station to say that Mrs. F is having difficulty breathing. You go into Mrs. F's room and assess the following: complaints of chest pain, R 36, P 110, coughing, dyspnea, anxiousness.

Instructions: On the basis of the situation **3 hours later**, identify and write the **priority problem** in the box below. Then, starting with the small box labeled **#1**, **prioritize** the **nursing interventions** for this situation and **identify** your follow-up action plan for Mrs. F.

NURSING INTERVENTIONS

A. Stay with Mrs. F

B. Raise head of bed

C. Take P, R, BP

D. Monitor oxygen saturation level

E. Notify MD

F. Administer oxygen

DECISION-MAKING DIAGRAM

New Action Plan

#1 #2 #3 #4 #5 #6

☐ ☐ ☐ ☐ ☐ ☐

Priority Problem

NOTES _____

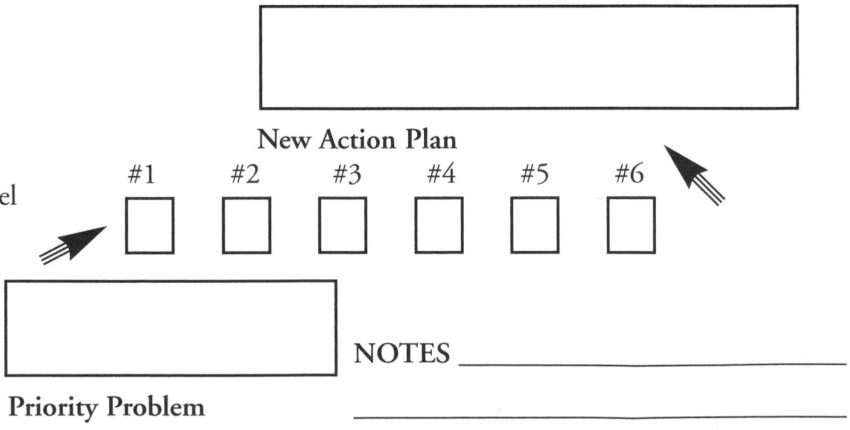

THE PATIENT WITH CIRRHOSIS OF THE LIVER

Mr. U, 46 years old, was admitted with the diagnosis of Laënnec's cirrhosis. In the evening report you learn that he is jaundiced, has ascites, and has increasing shortness of breath. His VS at 12:00 noon were T 99° F, P 94, R 34, BP 140/90. The vital signs are consistent with previous recordings. You get out of report at 4:30 PM. The nursing care Kardex (rand) includes the following orders:

VS q4h I & O (✓) Neuro cks q4h	Saline lock (✓)	Diet: ↑ CHO, 30 g Prot., 2 g Na^+
CBC, serum ammonia } today AST, ALT, PT	Bed rest with BRP	Routine med: Amphogel 30 mL po qid Furosemide 40 mg IV qAM Aldactone 50 mg po bid
Procedure: Abd. Paracentesis at 5:00 PM today	Weigh daily Measure abd girth daily	

TWO

Instructions: Prioritize the five **nursing interventions** as you would do them to take care of Mr. U. Write a number in the box to identify the order of your interventions (#1 = first intervention, #2 = second intervention, etc.) and state a **rationale** for each intervention.

INTERVENTIONS	PRIORITY #	RATIONALE
• Ensure that consent form is signed	☐	______
• Take the vital signs	☐	______
• Perform a body systems physical assessment	☐	______
• Ensure that abdominal paracentesis equipment is on the unit	☐	______
• Have Mr. U void	☐	______

KEY POINTS TO CONSIDER: ______________________

The physician performs the abdominal paracentesis on Mr. U and removes 2.5 L of fluid. VS during the procedure were P 90, R 32, BP 136/86. Post procedure you assess:

1. VS: P 94, R 24, BP 136/86
2. Dressing at the abdominal puncture site is clean
3. Mr. U is lying in a semi-Fowler's position
4. He is alert and oriented, although slow to respond

 Interactive activity: With a partner, **do the following:** (1) **select** the **one nursing diagnosis** that is of priority at this time, (2) **provide a rationale** for your selection, and (3) **list the nursing interventions** that assist to meet the needs of the patient.

All of the following nursing diagnoses may apply to Mr. U:

Risk for injury: Falls, Risk for infection, Impaired skin integrity, Risk for impaired physical mobility, Pain, Imbalanced nutrition: less than body requirements, Risk for disturbed thought processes, Risk for activity intolerance, Impaired tissue integrity, Excess fluid volume, Risk for deficient fluid volume, Ineffective breathing pattern, Disturbed body image, Disturbed sleep pattern, Fatigue, Altered comfort

Nursing Diagnosis	Rationale	Nursing Interventions

The **laboratory results** for today are:

PT 40 sec Serum ammonia 70 mcg/dL Hgb 10.6 g/dL Hct 30%
WBC 3500/mm^3 Platelets 100,000/mm^3 AST U/L ALT 500 U/L

Instructions: Based on the **laboratory results**, identify and write the **priority problem** in the box below. Then, starting with the small box labeled **#1, prioritize** the **nursing interventions** for this situation and **identify** your follow-up action plan for Mr. U.

NURSING INTERVENTIONS

A. Monitor the VS

B. Assess for petechiae

C. Check stool for occult blood

D. Monitor urine color

E. Check neuro status

F. Notify MD

DECISION-MAKING DIAGRAM

New Action Plan

#1 #2 #3 #4 #5 #6

☐ ☐ ☐ ☐ ☐ ☐

Priority Problem

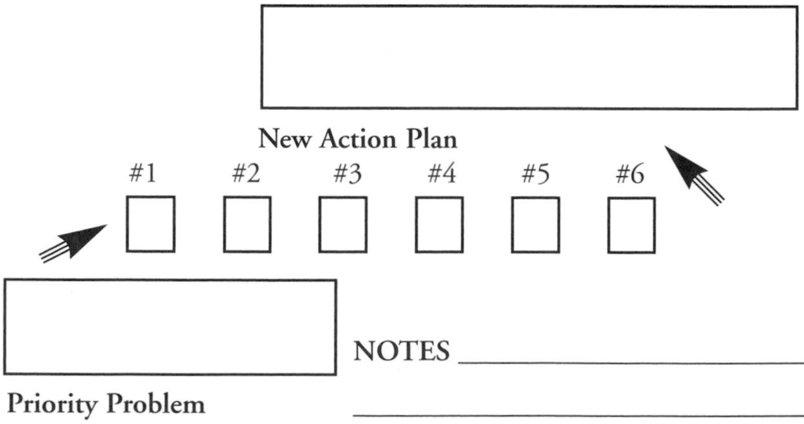

NOTES _____

APPLYING CRITICAL THINKING SKILLS TO TEST QUESTIONS

INSTRUCTIONS: Circle the one best answer for each test question. Write your rationale for selecting the answer. To enhance your learning and test-taking skills, discuss your answer and rationale with a partner. The answer and the rationale can be found on the back of this page.

1. The physicians order phytonadione (vitamin K) 10 mg IM for an adult client with liver cirrhosis and ascites. Available is a vial of phytonadione 10 mg/mL. The nurse is planning to administer this dose in the deltoid. Which of the following is most appropriate for the administration of the ordered amount to the client?
   a. 1-mL syringe with 25-gauge ⅝-inch needle
   b. 1-mL syringe with 23-gauge ½-inch needle
   c. 3-mL syringe with 23-gauge 1-inch needle
   d. 3-mL syringe with 22-gauge 1½-inch needle

   Rationale: ______________________________

2. The nurse admits a client with cirrhosis of the liver and severe ascites. The client is oriented, jaundiced, and complains of itching. Respirations are 28, short and shallow. Urine is dark amber. Which action is most important for the nurse to consider?
   a. Sit client in high-Fowler's position.
   b. Encourage client to drink more fluids.
   c. Limit client activity.
   d. Assess skin integrity daily.

   Rationale: ______________________________

3. The client is admitted with cirrhosis of the liver and ascites. The physician orders the administration of an IV infusion of albumin. Which of the following is the expected outcome after the administration of the albumin?
   a. Decreased complaints of pruritis
   b. Decreased serum ammonia levels
   c. Increased secretion of sodium
   d. Increased urinary output

   Rationale: ______________________________

TWO

ANSWER KEY FOR APPLYING CRITICAL THINKING SKILLS TO TEST QUESTIONS

HELPFUL HINTS: Read all test questions carefully. Identify key words in the question that will guide you in answering the question. In these test questions the **key words** to consider are **"most appropriate," "most important,"** and **"expected outcome."** Compare your rationale with the one in the test question.

1. The physicians order phytonadione (vitamin K) 10 mg IM for an adult client with liver cirrhosis and ascites. Available is a vial of phytonadione 10 mg/mL. The nurse is planning to administer this dose in the deltoid. Which of the following is most appropriate for the administration of the ordered amount to the client?
   a. 1-mL syringe with 25-gauge ⅝-inch needle
   b. 1-mL syringe with 23-gauge ½-inch needle
   (c.) 3-mL syringe with 23-gauge 1-inch needle
   d. 3-mL syringe with 22-gauge 1½-inch needle

   Rationale: The answer is (c). It is most appropriate to use a smaller IM needle gauge because clients with liver cirrhosis are at a high risk for bleeding. The deltoid is a smaller muscle than the gluteus, so a 1-inch needle is the best choice. Options (a), (b), and (d) are not the best choice for this client.

2. The nurse admits a client with cirrhosis of the liver and severe ascites. The client is oriented, jaundiced, and complains of itching. Respirations are 28, short and shallow. Urine is dark amber. Which action is most important for the nurse to consider?
   a. Sit client in high-Fowler's position.
   b. Encourage client to drink more fluids.
   (c.) Limit client activity.
   d. Assess skin integrity daily.

   Rationale: The answer is (c). Activity increases the metabolic needs of the body, thereby increasing the workload of the liver. Option (a) is not the most appropriate position for a client with severe ascites because it compromises respiration. Options (b) and (d) are not the most important interventions.

3. The client is admitted with cirrhosis of the liver and ascites. The physician orders the administration of an IV infusion of albumin. Which of the following is the expected outcome after the administration of the albumin?
   a. Decreased complaints of pruritis
   b. Decreased serum ammonia levels
   c. Increased secretion of sodium
   (d.) Increased urinary output

   Rationale: The answer is (d). Albumin increases plasma colloid osmotic pressure, thereby increasing diuresis. Options (a), (b), and (c) are not expected outcomes for this ordered intervention.

THE PATIENT WITH HEPATIC ENCEPHALOPATHY

Mr. U, 47 years old, is admitted with the diagnosis of hepatic encephalopathy related to his advanced cirrhosis of the liver. The night report indicates that he was awake most of the night and very restless during the shift. The nursing care Kardex has the following orders:

VS q4 I & O (✓) Neuro cks q4h Serum ammonia, K^+ today Code Status: No code	D_5W at 100 mL/hr #20 g RFA — inserted today Bed rest with BRP Weigh daily	Diet: ↑ CHO, 50 g Prot., 4 g Na^+ Routine med: Neomycin 1 g po q6h Lactulose 30 mL bid

TWO

As you enter his room you notice that Mr. U is sleeping.

Instructions: Prioritize the five **nursing interventions** as you would do them to take care of Mr. U. Write a number in the box to identify the order of your interventions (#1 = first intervention, #2 = second intervention, etc.) and state a **rationale** for each intervention.

INTERVENTIONS	PRIORITY #	RATIONALE
• Take VS	☐	______
• Assess the level of consciousness and orientation	☐	______
• Check current serum ammonia and K^+ levels	☐	______
• Perform a body systems physical assessment	☐	______
• Assist Mr. U with his activities of daily living	☐	______

KEY POINTS TO CONSIDER: ______

Mr. U has refused his morning dose of lactulose, and you further assess:

1. He refused the lactulose the previous day
2. No bowel movement for 2 days
3. Irritable, speech slurred
4. Responds slowly to verbal communication

Interactive activity: With a partner, **do the following:** (1) **select** the **one nursing diagnosis** that is of priority at this time, (2) **provide a rationale** for your selection, and (3) **list the nursing interventions** that assist to meet the needs of the patient.

All of the following nursing diagnoses may apply to Mr. U:

Risk for injury: falls, Risk for infection, Impaired skin integrity, Self-care deficit: bathing/hygiene, Risk for impaired physical mobility, Risk for constipation, Imbalanced nutrition: less than body requirements, Activity intolerance, Impaired tissue integrity, Excess fluid volume, Ineffective breathing pattern, Fatigue, Disturbed thought processes, Disturbed sleep pattern, Altered comfort

Nursing Diagnosis	Rationale	Nursing Interventions

You return from lunch at 1 PM and are informed of the following: Mr. U is becoming increasingly confused and lethargic. He did not eat lunch.

Instructions: Based on the 1 PM information, identify and write the **priority problem** in the box below. Then, starting with the small box labeled #1, **prioritize** the **nursing interventions** for this situation and **identify** your follow-up action plan for Mr. U.

NURSING INTERVENTIONS

A. Inform physician

B. Document assessment findings

C. Take VS

D. Monitor neurologic status

E. Stay with patient

F. Raise the bedrails

DECISION-MAKING DIAGRAM

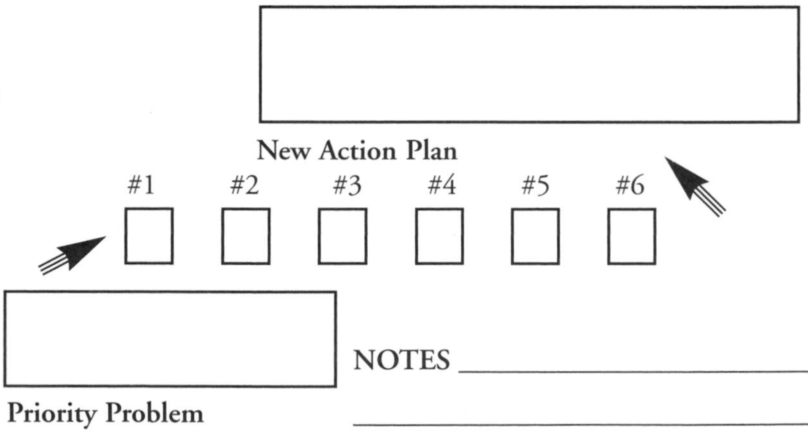

NOTES ______________________

____

APPLYING CRITICAL THINKING SKILLS TO TEST QUESTIONS

INSTRUCTIONS: Circle the one best answer for each test question. Write your rationale for selecting the answer. To enhance your learning and test-taking skills, discuss your answer and rationale with a partner. The answer and the rationale can be found on the back of this page.

TWO

1. The client is diagnosed with hepatic encephalopathy and is receiving lactulose 30 mL po bid. To effectively monitor the therapeutic effects of the drug therapy, the nurse would primarily assess for a(n):
   a. decrease in abdominal girth.
   b. increase in bowel movements.
   c. increase in serum albumin levels.
   d. decrease in serum ammonia levels.

   Rationale: ______________________________

2. The nurse administers spironolactone 100 mg po to a client with portal hypertension. Which of the following is most important for the nurse to monitor during the administration of this drug?
   a. Serum potassium levels
   b. Intake and output
   c. Specific gravity of urine
   d. Abdominal girth

   Rationale: ______________________________

3. The nurse is caring for a client admitted with portal hypertension and ascites. Which assessment finding is most indicative of a serious complication?
   a. Caput medusae noted on abdomen
   b. Complaints of fatigue and weakness
   c. Hematemesis after breakfast
   d. 2-pound weight loss from previous day

   Rationale: ______________________________

ANSWER KEY FOR APPLYING CRITICAL THINKING SKILLS TO TEST QUESTIONS

HELPFUL HINTS: Read all test questions carefully. Identify key words in the question that will guide you in answering the question. In these test questions the **key words** to consider are **"primarily," "most important,"** and **"most indicative."** Compare your rationale with the one in the test question.

1. The client is diagnosed with hepatic encephalopathy and is receiving lactulose 30 mL po bid. To effectively monitor the therapeutic effects of the drug therapy, the nurse would primarily assess for a(n):
   a. decrease in abdominal girth.
   b. increase in bowel movements.
   c. increase in serum albumin levels.
   (d.) decrease in serum ammonia levels.

   Rationale: The answer is (d). The expected therapeutic effect for this client is to decrease serum ammonia levels by trapping ammonium ions in the intestine and excreting them in the stool. Options (a) and (c) do not provide the nurse with a measure of the therapeutic drug effects, and option (b) is not as specific a measure of effectiveness as the serum ammonia level.

2. The nurse administers spironolactone 100 mg po to a client with portal hypertension. Which of the following is most important for the nurse to monitor during the administration of this drug?
   (a.) Serum potassium levels
   b. Intake and output
   c. Specific gravity of urine
   d. Abdominal girth

   Rationale: The answer is (a). Serum potassium levels should be monitored when a client is on spironolactone, a potassium-sparing diuretic. Options (b), (c), and (d) are not the most important interventions.

3. The nurse is caring for a client admitted with portal hypertension and ascites. Which assessment finding is most indicative of a serious complication?
   a. Caput medusae noted on abdomen
   b. Complaints of fatigue and weakness
   (c.) Hematemesis after breakfast
   d. 2-pound weight loss from previous day

   Rationale: The answer is (c). Clients with portal hypertension may also have esophageal varices. The client should be monitored for further signs of bleeding. Option (a) is an expected finding consistent with ascites. Option (b) needs further assessment, and option (d) is not most indicative of a serious complication.

THE PATIENT WITH DIABETES MELLITUS

The nurse is assigned to a 56-year-old Hispanic female, Mrs. G, admitted with the diagnosis of end-stage renal disease (ESRD). She has a 30-year history of type 1 diabetes mellitus. She is scheduled to have hemodialysis this AM. The night nurse indicates that she has a 2-cm dry, ulcerated circular area on the lateral outer aspect of her right great toe and an arteriovenous (AV) fistula in the right forearm. She has an order for NPH insulin 15 units Sub-Q qAM and blood glucose fingerstick ac and at 9:00 PM. It is 0730 when the nurse gets out of report, and breakfast arrives on the unit at 0800.

Instructions: Prioritize the five **nursing interventions** as you would do them to initially take care of Mrs. G. Write a number in the box to identify the order of your interventions (#1 = first intervention, #2 = second intervention, etc.) and state a **rationale** for each intervention.

INTERVENTIONS	PRIORITY #	RATIONALE
• Check chart for blood glucose fingerstick results	☐	__________
• Assess AV fistula	☐	__________
• Administer NPH 15 units Sub-Q	☐	__________
• Get patient ready for breakfast	☐	__________
• Perform a body systems physical assessment	☐	__________

KEY POINTS TO CONSIDER: __________

TWO

Mrs. G is still waiting for her dialysis treatment. At 1000 the physician leaves the following orders:

Sliding scale for fingerstick blood glucose: 225-250 units—give 10 units Reg insulin.
200-224 units—give 5 units Reg insulin.
150-199 units—give 2 units Reg insulin.
less than 150 units—no insulin

You do a fingerstick at 1130. The results are 236. You will give _______________ Regular insulin.

Interactive activity: With a partner, **do the following:** (1) **select** the **one nursing diagnosis** that is a priority at this time, (2) **provide a rationale** for your selection, and (3) **list the nursing interventions** that assist you to meet the needs of the patient.

All of the following nursing diagnoses may apply to Mrs. G:

Risk for infection, Risk for impaired skin integrity, Impaired physical mobility, Altered patterns of elimination, Ineffective sexuality patterns, Disturbed sensory perception, Fatigue, Excess fluid volume, Deficient fluid volume, Imbalanced nutrition: less than body requirements

Nursing Diagnosis	Rationale	Nursing Interventions

As you take her 1300 VS, you note the following signs and symptoms: Irritability, skin warm, moist, VS: T 36.8° C, P 100, R 18, BP 150/84. She complains of dizziness and "feeling funny." You suspect a hypoglycemic reaction.

Instructions: On the basis of the situation above, identify and write the **priority problem** in the box below. Then, starting with the small box labeled **#1**, **prioritize** the **nursing interventions** for this situation and **identify** your plan for follow-up care for Mrs. G.

NURSING INTERVENTIONS

A. Document findings/nursing care
B. Do a fingerstick blood glucose stat
C. Check fingerstick blood glucose in 15 minutes
D. Give 4 ounces of apple juice
E. Alert the RN stat
F. Raise the side rails

DECISION-MAKING DIAGRAM

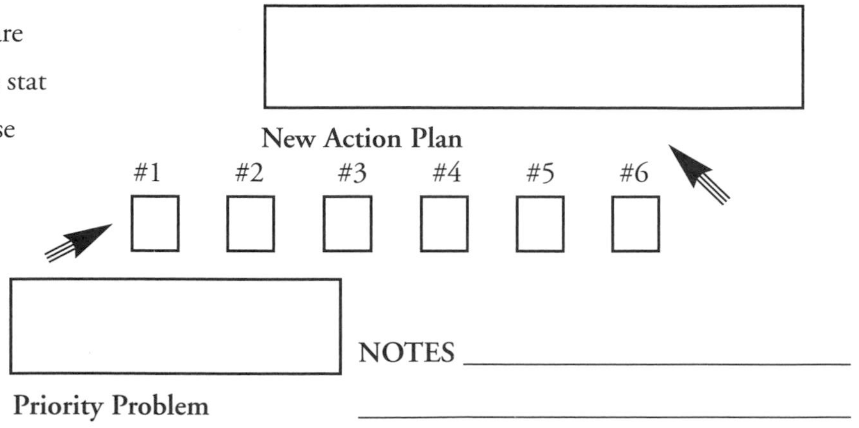

APPLYING CRITICAL THINKING SKILLS TO TEST QUESTIONS

INSTRUCTIONS: Circle the one best answer for each test question. Write your rationale for selecting the answer. To enhance your learning and test-taking skills, discuss your answer and rationale with a partner. The answer and the rationale can be found on the back of this page.

1. The nurse is providing discharge instructions to a newly diagnosed client with type 1 diabetes mellitus who will take 5 units Regular insulin and 10 units NPH insulin qAM. The client informs the nurse that he runs 2 miles every morning. In teaching the client about insulin absorption and exercise, it is important for the nurse to teach the client to:
   a. inject the morning dose of insulin into the abdomen.
   b. hold the morning dose of regular insulin until after the exercise.
   c. hold the morning dose of NPH insulin until after the exercise.
   d. inject the morning dose of insulin into the lower extremity.

   Rationale: ______________________________

2. The nurse notes the following medications on a client's medication record: NPH insulin 13 units Sub-Q qAM at 0730 and Humalog Lispro 5 units Sub-Q at the start of breakfast. The breakfast arrives at 0830 on the unit. In assessing the medication record, which action by the nurse is most appropriate?
   a. Question the Humalog Lispro insulin order.
   b. Question the NPH insulin order.
   c. Give both insulins at 0730 in one syringe.
   d. Give the insulins as ordered.

   Rationale: ______________________________

3. The nurse is preparing to draw up NPH 12 units using a low-dose insulin syringe. Which technique indicates the most appropriate procedure before giving the insulin? The nurse takes the medication record and the syringe with the 12 units of insulin and:
   a. checks the drawn-up dose with another nurse.
   b. with the syringe in the vial, checks the drawn-up dose with another nurse.
   c. takes the vial of insulin to check the drawn-up dose with another nurse.
   d. double checks by charting the dose of insulin before injecting the insulin.

   Rationale: ______________________________

ANSWER KEY FOR APPLYING CRITICAL THINKING SKILLS TO TEST QUESTIONS

HELPFUL HINTS: Read all test questions carefully. Identify key words in the question that will guide you in answering the question. In these test questions the **key words** to consider are "**absorption and exercise**" and "**most appropriate.**" Compare your rationale with the one in the test question.

1. The nurse is providing discharge instructions to a newly diagnosed client with type 1 diabetes mellitus who will take 5 units Regular insulin and 10 units NPH insulin qAM. The client informs the nurse that he runs 2 miles every morning. In teaching the client about insulin absorption and exercise, it is important for the nurse to teach the client to:
   - (a.) inject the morning dose of insulin into the abdomen. (circled)
   - b. hold the morning dose of regular insulin until after the exercise.
   - c. hold the morning dose of NPH insulin until after the exercise.
   - d. inject the morning dose of insulin into the lower extremity.

   Rationale: The answer is (a). The abdomen is a better injection site because the absorption rate of insulin is faster when injected into an extremity that is exercised. Options (b), (c), and (d) do not correlate the effects of diabetes, insulin therapy, and exercise.

2. The nurse notes the following medications on a client's medication record: NPH insulin 13 units Sub-Q qAM at 0730 and Humalog Lispro 5 units Sub-Q at the start of breakfast. The breakfast arrives at 0830 on the unit. In assessing the medication record, which action by the nurse is most appropriate?
   - a. Question the Humalog Lispro insulin order.
   - b. Question the NPH insulin order.
   - c. Give both insulins at 0730 in one syringe.
   - (d.) Give the insulins as ordered. (circled)

   Rationale: The answer is (d). It is most appropriate to consider that Humalog Lispro is a rapid-acting insulin with an onset of 10 to 15 minutes and should be administered at the start of the meal. Options (a), (b), and (c) do not address the onset of action of the rapid-acting insulin.

3. The nurse is preparing to draw up NPH 12 units using a low-dose insulin syringe. Which technique indicates the most appropriate procedure before giving the insulin? The nurse takes the medication record and the syringe with the 12 units of insulin and:
   - a. checks the drawn-up dose with another nurse.
   - (b.) with the syringe in the vial, checks the drawn-up dose with another nurse. (circled)
   - c. takes the vial of insulin to check the drawn-up dose with another nurse.
   - d. double checks by charting the dose of insulin before injecting the insulin.

   Rationale: The answer is (b). To prevent a medication error, it is recommended that the syringe remain in the insulin vial when checking the type and dose of insulin with another nurse. Options (a), (c), and (d) are not the most appropriate and recommended procedure.

THE PATIENT UNDERGOING HEMODIALYSIS

Ms. A, 52 years old, has ESRD and has just been started on dialysis. She has an AV fistula in the right forearm and is scheduled for dialysis at 0800 today. The night nurse reports that the fistula has a good thrill and bruit. Ms. A's BP is 160/102. You leave the report room at 0730 after noting the following orders from the nursing care Kardex:

VS q8h I & O (✓) Weigh daily Hgb & Hct, Serum ferritin (✓) Serum iron saturation (✓)	IV: Saline lock—left hand Routine medications: Vasotec 10 mg po qAM 0800 Folic acid 1 mg po qAM 0800 $FeSO_4$ 325 po tid c̄ meals Epogen 30,000 units Sub-Q M-W-F	Diet: 70 g Protein, 2 g Na^+, 2 g K^+ Fluid restriction 1000 mL/day

TWO

Instructions: Prioritize the five **nursing interventions** as you would do them to take care of Ms. A. Write a number in the box to identify the order of your interventions (#1 = first intervention, #2 = second intervention, etc.) and state a **rationale** for each intervention.

INTERVENTIONS	PRIORITY #	RATIONALE
• Take the VS (BP on the left arm)	☐	______
• Perform body systems physical assessment	☐	______
• Weigh patient/ensure patient has been weighed	☐	______
• Assess AV fistula for thrill and bruit	☐	______
• Hold folic acid and Vasotec	☐	______

KEY POINTS TO CONSIDER: ______

Ordered laboratory studies were drawn before dialysis. The results of the morning laboratory tests are:

1. Hemoglobin 9.5 g/dL, hematocrit 28%
2. Ferritin 60 ng/L
3. Serum iron saturation 18%
4. K^+ 5.0 mEq

Interactive activity: With a partner, **do the following:** (1) **select** the **one nursing diagnosis** that is of priority at this time, (2) **provide a rationale** for your selection, and (3) **list the nursing interventions** that assist to meet the needs of the patient.

All of the following nursing diagnoses may apply to Ms. A:

Risk for injury, Deficient knowledge, Fear, Anxiety, Risk for infection, Impaired tissue integrity, Risk for disturbed sensory perception, Constipation, Excess fluid volume, Deficient fluid volume, Disturbed body image, Risk for impaired physical mobility, Ineffective tissue perfusion, Imbalanced nutrition: less than body requirements, Fatigue

Nursing Diagnosis	Rationale	Nursing Interventions

After the dialysis treatment, Ms. A is restless and you assess: Complains of headache, pruritus, nausea, change in level of consciousness, twitching, confusion

Instructions: On the basis of data **after the dialysis treatment data**, identify and write the **priority problem** in the box below. Then, starting with the small box labeled **#1**, **prioritize** the **nursing interventions** for this situation and **identify** your follow-up action plan for Ms. A.

NURSING INTERVENTIONS

A. Take the VS

B. Notify physician

C. Maintain calm, quiet environment

D. Stay with patient

E. Monitor neurologic status

F. Document assessment findings

DECISION-MAKING DIAGRAM

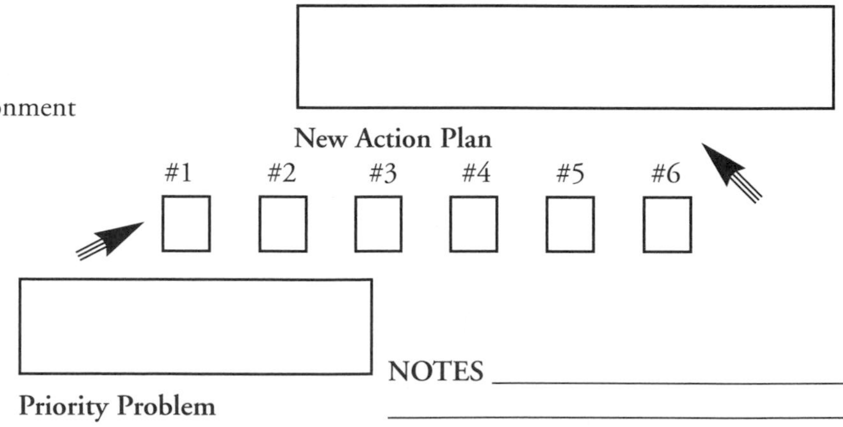

NOTES

APPLYING CRITICAL THINKING SKILLS TO TEST QUESTIONS

INSTRUCTIONS: Circle the one best answer for each test question. Write your rationale for selecting the answer. To enhance your learning and test-taking skills, discuss your answer and rationale with a partner. The answer and the rationale can be found on the back of this page.

1. The client with ESRD related to type 1 diabetes mellitus has completed hemodialysis 1 hour ago. Which nursing intervention is of priority in assisting the alert adult client to transfer from the bed to the chair after dialysis?
   a. Check the blood glucose level.
   b. Monitor for dizziness on standing.
   c. Wrap the AV fistula with gauze.
   d. Do not move the arm with the AV fistula.

   Rationale: ____

2. The nurse administers epoetin10,000 units Sub-Q twice weekly to the client with ESRD. The most effective method of evaluating the therapeutic effect of epoetin is for the nurse to assess for:
   a. a decrease in skin pallor.
   b. an increase in client activity.
   c. an increase in the hematocrit level.
   d. a decrease in complaints of weakness and fatigue.

   Rationale: ____

3. The nurse is caring for a client scheduled for hemodialysis this morning. In preparing the client for the dialysis treatment, it is most important for the nurse to:
   a. allow the client to rest until after the dialysis treatment.
   b. ensure that all morning care is completed before dialysis.
   c. make the client NPO until after the dialysis treatment.
   d. withhold the morning dose of any antihypertensive drugs.

   Rationale: ____

TWO

ANSWER KEY FOR APPLYING CRITICAL THINKING SKILLS TO TEST QUESTIONS

HELPFUL HINTS: Read all test questions carefully. Identify key words in the question that will guide you in answering the question. In these test questions the **key words** to consider are "**priority,**" "**most effective,**" and "**most important.**" Compare your rationale with the one in the test question.

1. The client with ESRD related to type 1 diabetes mellitus has completed hemodialysis 1 hour ago. Which nursing intervention is of priority in assisting the alert adult client to transfer from the bed to the chair after dialysis?
   a. Check the blood glucose level.
   (b.) Monitor for dizziness on standing.
   c. Wrap the AV fistula with gauze.
   d. Do not move the arm with the AV fistula.

   Rationale: The answer is (b). Hypotension is a postdialysis complication related to rapid removal of fluid. The nurse should monitor for orthostatic changes. Options (a) and (c) are important but not of priority after dialysis. Option (d) is an intervention that can apply to a new fistula.

2. The nurse administers epoetin10,000 units Sub-Q twice weekly to the client with ESRD. The most effective method of evaluating the therapeutic effect of epoetin is for the nurse to assess for:
   a. a decrease in skin pallor.
   b. an increase in client activity.
   (c.) an increase in the hematocrit level.
   d. a decrease in complaints of weakness and fatigue.

   Rationale: The answer is (c). Epoetin stimulates the production of red blood cells. The hematocrit is an indirect measurement of the total number and volume of red blood cells. Options (a), (b), and (d) may be manifested as a result of the rise in the number of red blood cells.

3. The nurse is caring for a client scheduled for hemodialysis this morning. In preparing the client for the dialysis treatment, it is most important for the nurse to:
   a. allow the client to rest until after the dialysis treatment.
   b. ensure that all morning care is completed before dialysis.
   c. make the client NPO until after the dialysis treatment.
   (d.) withhold the morning dose of any antihypertensive drugs.

   Rationale: The answer is (d). Hypotension is a complication of dialysis. Antihypertensive drugs taken before dialysis can cause severe hypotension. Options (a) and (b) are not the most important in preparing the client, and option (c) is not necessary in preparing the client for hemodialysis.

THE PATIENT WITH PERIPHERAL ARTERIAL DISEASE

Mr. L, 70 years old, is sent to the hospital after visiting his physician with complaints of increasing painful muscle cramps after ambulating. He lives alone, and his medical history is significant for hypertension.

The nursing care Kardex has the following admission orders:

VS q4h I & O (✓) Pedal pulse check q4h Bed rest with BRP CBC Mr. L Age: 70	Insert saline lock Drsg chgs: Clean ulcerated area on left foot with NS—apply dry sterile 4 × 4s Dx. Peripheral arterial disease	Diet: Mech Soft Routine med: Trental 400 mg po tid Dipyridamole 50 mg po tid

TWO

You are assigned to begin his admission. You note that he is alert but hard of hearing. He has a bandage around his left foot. He tells you he uses this to keep his shoe from rubbing his foot.

Instructions: Prioritize the five **nursing interventions** as you would do them to take care of Mr. L. Write a number in the box to identify the order of your interventions (#1 = first intervention, #2 = second intervention, etc.) and state a **rationale** for each intervention.

INTERVENTIONS	PRIORITY #	RATIONALE
• Take the VS	☐	______
• Assess bilateral pedal pulses	☐	______
• Orient to hospital room	☐	______
• Perform a body systems assessment	☐	______
• Apply sterile dressing to left foot	☐	______

KEY POINTS TO CONSIDER: ______

You assist Mr. L to the bathroom; on his return to bed you note the following:

1. Bilateral lower extremities—reddish blue in color
2. Bilateral pedal pulses weak (1+), capillary refill >3 seconds
3. Lower extremities cool to touch
4. Gait slow, needs assistance

Interactive activity: With a partner, **do the following:** (1) **select** the **one nursing diagnosis** that is of priority at this time, (2) **provide a rationale** for your selection, and (3) **list the nursing interventions** that assist to meet the needs of the patient.

All of the following nursing diagnoses may apply to Mr. L:

Risk for injury: fall, Deficient knowledge, Risk for infection, Impaired skin integrity, Self-care deficit, Risk for impaired physical mobility, Ineffective peripheral tissue perfusion, Activity intolerance, Impaired tissue integrity, Pain

Nursing Diagnosis	Rationale	Nursing Interventions

You **remove the bandage** from the left foot and you note: A circular ulcerated area with two toes blackened and shriveled

Instructions: On the basis of **removal of the bandage** information, identify and write the **priority problem** in the box below. Then, starting with the small box labeled #1, **prioritize** the **nursing interventions** for this situation and **identify** your follow-up action plan for Mr. L.

NURSING INTERVENTIONS

A. Assess pain level
B. Measure ulcerated area
C. Apply sterile gloves
D. Cleanse area with normal saline solution
E. Apply sterile dressing
F. Document assessment findings

DECISION-MAKING DIAGRAM

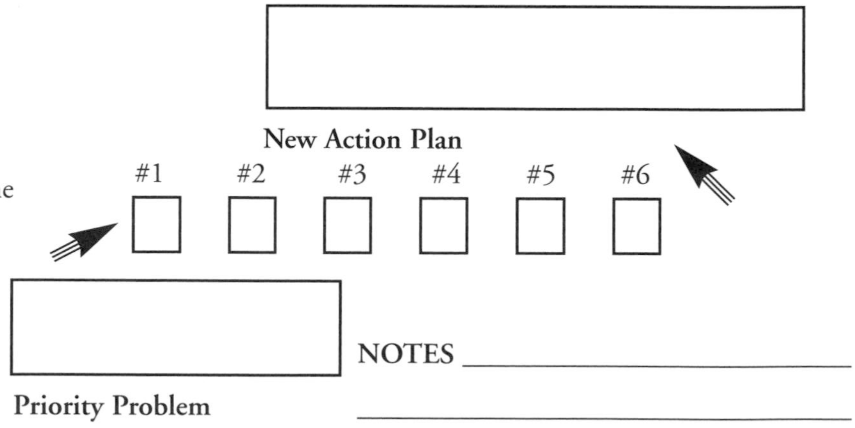

THE PATIENT WITH CHEST PAIN

Mrs. T, 56 years old, was admitted after having chest pain. She has coronary artery disease and smokes 1 pack of cigarettes a day. Her father died of heart disease and she has a brother with hypertension. Her VS are T 98° F, P 90, R 26, BP 164/100. Mrs. T has been taking verapamil, Procardia, and Tenormin. Mrs. T will continue with her usual cardiac and blood pressure medications and is also started on aspirin 81 mg, Colace, and Lovastatin. Nitroglycerin tablets 0.4 mg SL is ordered prn chest pain and Mylanta 30 mL q2h prn. She has bathroom privileges with assistance, a saline lock, and oxygen at 2-3 L/nasal cannula to keep the oxygen saturation >96%. The night nurse reports that Mrs. T is upset about not being able to smoke. Mrs. T is requesting to use the commode as you start your shift.

TWO

Instructions: Prioritize the five **nursing interventions** as you would do them to initially take care of Mrs. T. Write a number in the box to identify the order of your interventions (#1 = first intervention, #2 = second intervention, etc.) and state a **rationale** for each intervention.

INTERVENTIONS	PRIORITY #	RATIONALE
• Take the vital signs	☐	______
• Assist to commode	☐	______
• Perform a body systems assessment	☐	______
• Check oxygen saturation level	☐	______
• Talk with Mrs. T	☐	______

KEY POINTS TO CONSIDER: ______

______

______

After breakfast Mrs. T continues to be upset. She states that she is constipated and above all wants to smoke. She is getting increasingly upset. You observe the following:

1. Abdomen round, bowel sounds present in all four quadrants
2. Breakfast intake 30%
3. Last bowel movement 2 days ago
4. O_2 saturation at 93%

Interactive activity: With a partner, **do the following:** (1) **select** the **one nursing diagnosis** that is of priority at this time, (2) **provide a rationale** for your selection, and (3) **list the nursing interventions** that assist to meet the needs of the patient.

All of the following nursing diagnoses may apply to Mrs. T:

Pain, Deficient knowledge, Anxiety, Risk for noncompliance, Risk for decreased cardiac output, Activity intolerance, Ineffective tissue perfusion: cardiopulmonary, Risk for impaired skin integrity, Constipation, Ineffective health maintenance

Nursing Diagnosis	Rationale	Nursing Interventions

At **10:00 AM** the nursing assistant reports that Mrs. T is experiencing chest pain. You assess and note that she has cool, clammy skin, complains of tightness in the chest with pain radiating to the left arm, BP 154/98, P 100, R 30. Oxygen is at 2 L/nasal cannula, oxygen saturation is 88%.

Instructions: On the basis of the data at **10:00 AM**, identify and write the **priority problem** in the box below. Then, starting with the small box labeled **#1**, **prioritize** the **nursing interventions** for this situation and **identify** your follow-up action plan for Mrs. T.

NURSING INTERVENTIONS

A. Increase oxygen

B. Prepare to give morphine sulfate, if ordered

C. Administer nitroglycerin tab i q5min × 3

D. Monitor VS q5min

E. Obtain 12-lead electrocardiogram per protocol

F. Notify physician

DECISION-MAKING DIAGRAM

New Action Plan

#1 #2 #3 #4 #5 #6

Priority Problem

NOTES ______________________

THE PATIENT WITH HEART FAILURE

You are assigned to Mr. T, who was transferred to your unit earlier today. In report you learn that he has heart failure (HF), 3+ pitting edema of the lower extremities, increasing shortness of breath, and has been demonstrating Cheyne-Stokes respirations and periods of confusion; he complains of blurred vision. Vital signs are T 97.6° F, P 62, R 22, BP 180/102. He has received his 0900 meds. Current orders include:

VS q4h I & O (✓) Up in chair QID O_2 @ 3L/NP Serum K^+, PT, PTT, ABG (✓) Chest x-ray (✓) ECG (✓) Name: T. Age: 72	IV D5W @ 50 mL/hr IV site: LFA #20 g LBM: 2 days ago Foley (✓) Code Status: Full code Dx: HF	Diet: Soft (NAS) Routine medications: Digoxin 0.25 mg IV qAM 0900 Furosemide 40 mg po bid 0900-1700 Docusate sodium tab i po qAM 0900 Minipress 10 mg po bid 0900-1700

Instructions: Prioritize the five **nursing interventions** as you would do them to take care of Mr. T. Write a number in the box to identify the order of your interventions (#1 = first intervention, #2 = second intervention, etc.) and state a **rationale** for each intervention.

INTERVENTIONS	PRIORITY #	RATIONALE
• Assess respiratory rate	☐	
• Obtain urinary output data	☐	
• Assess rate/rhythm and quality of pulse	☐	
• Assess complaints of visual disturbances	☐	
• Check current lab data	☐	

KEY POINTS TO CONSIDER:

TWO

Mr. T wants to wash up, but he says that he does not have the energy like he used to and that he gets tired very easily. You assess the following:

1. Skin cool, dusky in color
2. Lower extremities with 2+ pitting edema
3. Lung sounds with crackles on inspiration; R 24, regular pattern
4. Alert and oriented at this time

Interactive activity: With a partner, **do the following:** (1) **select** the **one nursing diagnosis** that is of priority at this time, (2) **provide a rationale** for your selection, and (3) **list the nursing interventions** that assist you to meet the needs of the patient.

All of the following nursing diagnoses may apply to Mr. T:

Anxiety, Risk for infection, Activity intolerance, Excess fluid volume, Impaired tissue integrity, Risk for ineffective tissue perfusion: cerebral, Imbalanced nutrition: less than body requirements, Risk for injury, Deficient knowledge, Impaired gas exchange, Fatigue

Nursing Diagnosis	Rationale	Nursing Interventions

Mr. T's family stops to visit during lunch. **At 1:00 PM**, the nursing assistant tells you that Mr. T is in distress. You walk into the room and notice Mr. T holding his chest tightly. Shortly after, you assess: cyanosis, no pulse, no BP, and no respirations.

Instructions: On the basis of the situation at **1:00 PM**, identify and write the **priority problem** in the box below. Then, starting with the small box labeled **#1**, **prioritize** the **nursing interventions** for this situation and **identify** your follow-up action plan for Mr. T.

NURSING INTERVENTIONS

A. Call a code
B. Place in supine position
C. Begin CPR
D. Notify physician
E. Document findings
F. Support family

DECISION-MAKING DIAGRAM

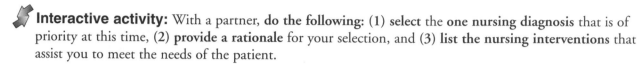

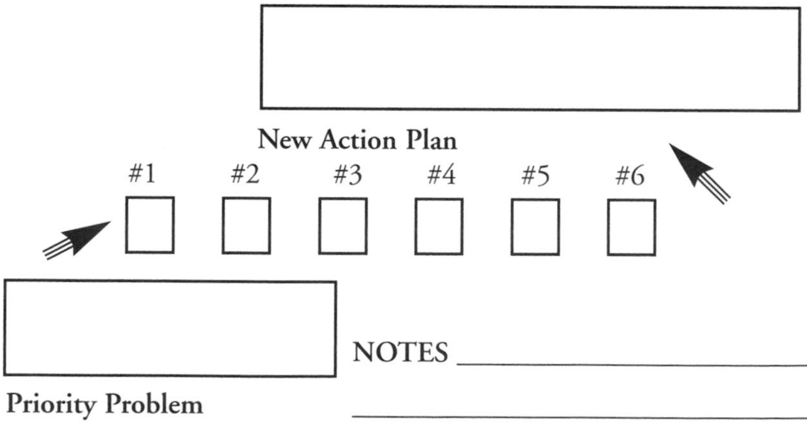

NOTES ______________________

____

For a continuation of this case study, go to *http://evolve.elsevier.com/castillo/thinking.*

APPLYING CRITICAL THINKING SKILLS TO TEST QUESTIONS

INSTRUCTIONS: Circle the one best answer for each test question. Write your rationale for selecting the answer. To enhance your learning and test-taking skills, discuss your answer and rationale with a partner. The answer and the rationale can be found on the back of this page.

1. The nurse admits a 69-year-old male client with HF. The physician orders furosemide 60 mg IV stat, digoxin 0.25 mg po, and KCl 20 mEq po now. Which assessment finding is most indicative of an ineffective response 2 hours after the administration of all the medications?
   a. Pulse 89, irregular
   b. Urine output 60 mL
   c. Pulse oximetry 94%
   d. Pitting edema in the lower extremities

   Rationale: ____

2. The home health nurse visits a client with HF. In reviewing the client's medications, the nurse notes that the client takes the following daily oral medications: digoxin 0.25 mg, furosemide 10 mg, and captopril 0.625 mg. After speaking to the client and wife, the nurse suspects digitalis toxicity. Which question helps the nurse gather more information specific to digitalis toxicity?
   a. "Do you get light-headed when you get out of bed?"
   b. "Do you need to sleep with more than one pillow?"
   c. "Do you have to get up to urinate more frequently?"
   d. "Have you had any nausea, vomiting, or diarrhea?"

   Rationale: ____

3. The nurse is assigned to a client with HF. The nurse's morning lung assessment indicates crackles and wheezes in the mid to lower lung bases, R 32, client restless. Which nursing intervention is of priority initially?
   a. Assess capillary refill
   b. Take the pulse oximetry
   c. Limit client activity
   d. Assess fluid intake

   Rationale: ____

ANSWER KEY FOR APPLYING CRITICAL THINKING SKILLS TO TEST QUESTIONS

HELPFUL HINTS: Read all test questions carefully. Identify key words in the question that will guide you in answering the question. In these test questions the **key words** to consider are "**most indicative,**" "**specific information,**" and "**priority initially.**" Compare your rationale with the one in the test question.

1. The nurse admits a 69-year-old male client with HF. The physician orders furosemide 60 mg IV stat, digoxin 0.25 mg po, and KCl 20 mEq po now. Which assessment finding is most indicative of an ineffective response 2 hours after the administration of all the medications?
   a. Pulse 89, irregular
   (b.) Urine output 60 mL
   c. Pulse oximetry 94%
   d. Pitting edema in the lower extremities

   Rationale: The answer is (b). Although output falls within the parameters of renal function, the client received furosemide IV and diuresis is the desired effect. Options (a), (c), and (d) are expected findings in a client with HF.

2. The home health nurse visits a client with HF. In reviewing the client's medications, the nurse notes that the client takes the following daily oral medications: digoxin 0.25 mg, furosemide 10 mg, and captopril 0.625 mg. After speaking to the client and wife, the nurse suspects digitalis toxicity. Which question helps the nurse gather more information specific to digitalis toxicity?
   a. "Do you get light-headed when you get out of bed?"
   b. "Do you need to sleep with more than one pillow?"
   c. "Do you have to get up to urinate more frequently?"
   (d.) "Have you had any nausea, vomiting, or diarrhea?"

   Rationale: The answer is (d). Although these signs and symptoms are frequently seen with all drug therapy, they are frequently early side effects of digitalis toxicity. Options (a), (b), and (c) relate to the action of the other drugs.

3. The nurse is assigned to a client with HF. The nurse's morning lung assessment indicates crackles and wheezes in the mid to lower lung bases, R 32, client restless. Which nursing intervention is of priority initially?
   a. Assess capillary refill
   (b.) Take the pulse oximetry
   c. Limit client activity
   d. Assess fluid intake

   Rationale: The answer is (b). Client assessment indicates rapid breathing and possible hypoxia. To fully assess the respiratory status of the client, it is important to take the pulse oximetry. Options (a), (c), and (d) are important—but not priority—interventions.

THE PATIENT WITH A STROKE

Mr. H, 68 years old, has had a right-sided stroke. He was admitted to the telemety unit 2 days ago and he has been on heparin therapy. The latest documentation in the nursing notes shows: Hand grips R > L, speech slurred, BP 166/102. The orders in the nursing care Kardex include the following:

VS q4h I & O (✓) Neuro checks q4h Up in chair today O_2 @ 2L/NP Hospital day: #3	IV: 500 mL: D5W/with heparin 10,000 units infuse at 1000 units/hr Foley (✓) Foley care bid ROM to Left side Serum K^+, Na^+ & CBC today PTT daily	Diet: Full liquid Swallowing precautions Routine med: Docusate sodium 20 mg (5 mL) po bid Nimodipine 20 mg po tid

You begin your shift and during report you learn that Mr. H had a restful night and there were no changes in his condition. You prepare to assist Mr. H with his breakfast.

Instructions: Prioritize the five **nursing interventions** as you would do them to take care of Mr. H. Write a number in the box to identify the order of your interventions (#1 = first intervention, #2 = second intervention, etc.) and state a **rationale** for each intervention.

INTERVENTIONS	PRIORITY #	RATIONALE
• Place in high-Fowler's position	☐	
• Place food on right side for patient to see	☐	
• Place food into unaffected side of mouth	☐	
• Check inside of mouth for food caught between gums and teeth (pocketing)	☐	
• Use thickened liquids	☐	

KEY POINTS TO CONSIDER:

TWO

As morning care is given to Mr. H, you assess the following:

1. Does not turn head if spoken to from left side
2. Left hand/arm elevated on a pillow
3. Passive range of motion is performed to extremities on the left side
4. Antiembolic stockings on
5. Lack of awareness of left side

 Interactive activity: With a partner, **do the following: (1) select the one nursing diagnosis** that is of priority at this time, **(2) provide a rationale** for your selection, and **(3) list the nursing interventions** that assist you to meet the needs of the patient.

All of the following nursing diagnoses may apply to Mr. H:

> Risk for injury: Falls, Deficient knowledge, Fear, Anxiety, Risk for infection, Impaired tissue integrity, Disturbed sensory perception, Constipation, Impaired swallowing, Impaired verbal communication, Self-care deficit: bathing/hygiene, Impaired urinary elimination, Disturbed body image, Risk for impaired physical mobility, Ineffective tissue perfusion, Unilateral neglect, Risk for aspiration, Risk for disuse syndrome

Nursing Diagnosis	Rationale	Nursing Interventions

Mr. H's laboratory data are called to the unit. The results are as follows: PTT 250 sec (control 38 sec), K^+ 3.5 mEq, Na^+ 145 mEq, Hgb 11.4 g/dL, Hct 34%, platelets 110,000/mm^3

Instructions: Based on **Mr. H's laboratory** data, identify and write the **priority problem** in the box below. Then, starting with the small box labeled **#1, prioritize** the **nursing interventions** for this situation and **identify** your follow-up action plan for Mr. H.

NURSING INTERVENTIONS

A. Notify physician

B. Prepare to administer protamine sulfate (if ordered)

C. Assess for petechiae

D. Monitor urine color

E. Monitor neuro status

F. Take the VS

DECISION-MAKING DIAGRAM

New Action Plan

#1 #2 #3 #4 #5 #6

□ □ □ □ □ □

Priority Problem

NOTES _____

APPLYING CRITICAL THINKING SKILLS TO TEST QUESTIONS

INSTRUCTIONS: Circle the one best answer for each test question. Write your rationale for selecting the answer. To enhance your learning and test-taking skills, discuss your answer and rationale with a partner. The answer and the rationale can be found on the back of this page.

1. The nurse is caring for a client who had a right-sided stroke 5 days ago and is experiencing unilateral neglect. In delegating the care of the client, which nursing intervention is of priority? The nurse instructs the nursing assistant to:
   a. have the client use a communication board.
   b. place the food tray to the right side of the body.
   c. remind the client to look at the left side of the body.
   d. provide passive range of motion to the left side of the body.

   Rationale: ____________________

2. The nurse walks into a client's room. The client is in low Fowler's position and the wife is feeding him small amounts of applesauce. The client had a left-sided stroke 7 days ago, is on a dysphagic diet, and has an indwelling urinary catheter. Which nursing action is of priority for this client?
   a. Raise the head of the bed.
   b. Encourage the wife to talk softly to the client.
   c. Remind the client to look and touch the affected side.
   d. Assess the color and amount of output.

   Rationale: ____________________

3. The nurse is preparing to administer oral medications to a client who is on a dysphagic diet. Which nursing action is best in administering the medications to the client? Crush the medications and:
   a. put the crushed medications in 15 mL of tap water.
   b. mix the crushed medications in 4 oz of applesauce.
   c. dissolve the crushed medications in 30 mL of warm water.
   d. mix the crushed medications in 30 mL of thickened liquid.

   Rationale: ____________________

ANSWER KEY FOR APPLYING CRITICAL THINKING SKILLS TO TEST QUESTIONS

HELPFUL HINTS: Read all test questions carefully. Identify key words in the question that will guide you in answering the question. In these test questions the **key words** to consider are "**priority**" and "**best.**" Compare your rationale with the one in the test question.

1. The nurse is caring for a client who had a right-sided stroke 5 days ago and is experiencing unilateral neglect. In delegating the care of the client, which nursing intervention is of priority? The nurse instructs the nursing assistant to:
   a. have the client use a communication board.
   b. place the food tray to the right side of the body.
   (c.) remind the client to look at the left side of the body.
   d. provide passive range of motion to the left side of the body.

   Rationale: The answer is (c). Clients who have a right-sided stroke have spatial and perceptual deficits. Clients will neglect the left side of the body. Options (a), (b), and (d) do not correlate the clients need to the intervention.

2. The nurse walks into a client's room. The client is in low Fowler's position and the wife is feeding him small amounts of applesauce. The client had a left-sided stroke 7 days ago, is on a dysphagic diet, and has an indwelling urinary catheter. Which nursing action is of priority for this client?
   (a.) Raise the head of the bed.
   b. Encourage the wife to talk softly to the client.
   c. Remind the client to look and touch the affected side.
   d. Assess the color and amount of output.

   Rationale: The answer is (a). The potential for aspiration is a serious concern. Every nursing measure should be implemented to prevent this complication. Options (b), (c), and (d) are important, but they are not priorities at this time.

3. The nurse is preparing to administer oral medications to a client who is on a dysphagic diet. Which nursing action is best in administering the medications to the client? Crush the medications and:
   a. put the crushed medications in 15 mL of tap water.
   b. mix the crushed medications in 4 oz of applesauce.
   c. dissolve the crushed medications in 30 mL of warm water.
   (d.) mix the crushed medications in 30 mL of thickened liquid.

   Rationale: The answer is (d). Use a small amount of thickened liquids to mix and administer the medications. Options (a) and (c) are not appropriate because water may cause the client to aspirate. Option (b) is mixing the medications in too large a quantity of applesauce.

THE PATIENT WITH CHRONIC OBSTRUCTIVE PULMONARY DISEASE

You are assigned to Mr. Y, a 61-year-old man who has chronic obstructive pulmonary disease (COPD). In the morning report you learn that he has been agitated during the night and is dyspneic this morning. The 0600 vital signs are T 98.8° F, P 102, R 32, BP 146/98. His 0700 pulse oximeter reading was 89% (room air) and he has an aminophylline drip infusing at 6 mg/hr per pump and oxygen at 2 L/nasal cannula. He receives albuterol inhaler 2 puffs q4h and Atrovent inhaler 2 puffs q4h. He had a serum theophylline level drawn in the evening. It is now 0730.

Instructions: Prioritize the five **nursing interventions** as you would do them to initially take care of Mr. Y. Write a number in the box to identify the order of your interventions (#1 = first intervention, #2 = second intervention, etc.) and state a **rationale** for each intervention.

INTERVENTIONS	PRIORITY #	RATIONALE
• Auscultate lung sounds	☐	______
• Assess pulse oximeter, oxygen, and nasal cannula	☐	______
• Retake the vital signs	☐	______
• Check theophylline level	☐	______
• Place in high-Fowler's position	☐	______

KEY POINTS TO CONSIDER: ______

______

______

TWO

As you provide morning care to Mr. Y, you note the following signs and symptoms:
1. Nonproductive cough; long expiratory phase during respiration
2. Increased shortness of breath with mild exertion
3. Crackles audible throughout the bilateral lung fields
4. Anxious and restless
5. Theophylline level 14 mcg/mL

Interactive activity: With a partner, **do the following:** (1) **select** the **one nursing diagnosis** that is of priority at this time, (2) **provide a rationale** for your selection, and (3) **list the nursing interventions** that assist to meet the needs of the patient.

All of the following nursing diagnoses may apply to Mr. Y:

> Ineffective breathing pattern, Ineffective airway clearance, Risk for injury, Risk for infection, Anxiety, Impaired gas exchange, Activity intolerance, Risk for impaired skin integrity, Imbalanced nutrition: less than body requirements, Sexual dysfunction

Nursing Diagnosis	Rationale	Nursing Interventions

At **12:00 noon** the patient care assistant reports that Mr. Y is very warm and that his VS are T 102° F, P 98, R 32, BP 140/84. He is expectorating thick, yellow-colored sputum.

Instructions: Based on the situation at **12:00 noon**, identify and write the **priority problem** in the box below. Then, starting with the small box labeled **#1**, **prioritize** the **nursing interventions** for this situation and **identify** your follow-up action plan for Mr. Y.

NURSING INTERVENTIONS DECISION-MAKING DIAGRAM

A. Auscultate lung sounds

B. Administer antipyretic if ordered

C. Provide cooling measures

D. Check oxygen saturation level

E. Retake VS in 2 hr

F. Inform physician

New Action Plan

#1 #2 #3 #4 #5 #6

☐ ☐ ☐ ☐ ☐ ☐

Priority Problem

NOTES _____

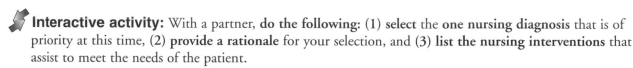

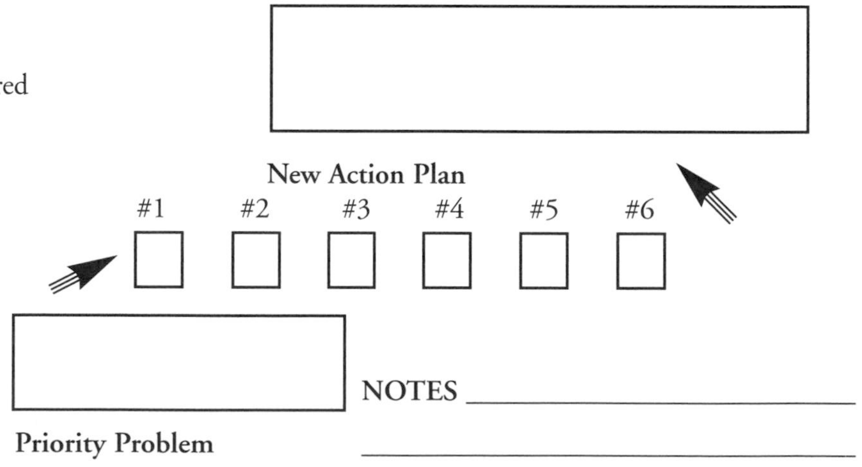

APPLYING CRITICAL THINKING SKILLS TO TEST QUESTIONS

INSTRUCTIONS: **Circle the one best answer for each test question.** Write your rationale for selecting the answer. To enhance your learning and test-taking skills, discuss your answer and rationale with a partner. The answer and the rationale can be found on the back of this page.

1. The nurse is caring for a client who was admitted with an exacerbation of COPD. The client's respirations are 28 with dyspnea on exertion. The client is receiving 2 L of oxygen per nasal cannula. The morning pulse oximetry is 92%. Which nursing intervention is of priority?
   a. Monitor the client.
   b. Notify the physician.
   c. Get an order to increase the oxygen.
   d. Place in semi-Fowler's position.

   Rationale: ____________________

2. The client has a long history of COPD and is currently experiencing an exacerbation of COPD. The following lab work is done this morning: complete blood cell count, arterial blood gases, and an electrolyte panel consisting of K^+, Na^+, Cl^-, carbon dioxide, blood urea nitrogen, and fasting blood glucose. Which laboratory data will require immediate follow-up?
   a. PaO_2 WNL
   b. Increased RBCs
   c. Increased $PaCO_2$
   d. Hgb WNL

   Rationale: ____________________

3. The client is admitted with an acute exacerbation of COPD. Which assessment finding is most indicative of a potential complication?
   a. R 32, increasingly anxious and restless
   b. Using accessory muscles during respiration
   c. Pulse oximetry 92%, pursed-lip breathing
   d. Expectorating copious amount of white phlegm

   Rationale: ____________________

TWO

ANSWER KEY FOR APPLYING CRITICAL THINKING SKILLS TO TEST QUESTIONS

HELPFUL HINTS: Read all test questions carefully. Identify key words in the question that will guide you in answering the question. In these test questions the **key words** to consider are "**priority,**" "**immediate,**" and "**most indicative.**" Compare your rationale with the one in the test question.

1. The nurse is caring for a client who was admitted with an exacerbation of COPD. The client's respirations are 28 with dyspnea on exertion. The client is receiving 2 L of oxygen per nasal cannula. The morning pulse oximetry is 92%. Which nursing intervention is of priority?
   (a.) Monitor the client.
   b. Notify the physician.
   c. Get an order to increase the oxygen.
   d. Place in semi-Fowler's position.

   Rationale: The answer is (a). The client is manifesting signs and symptoms consistent with COPD. Clients with COPD experience some degree of hypoxia. Options (b) and (c) are not appropriate at this time. Option (d) is not the best position for a client with COPD.

2. The client has a long history of COPD and is currently experiencing an exacerbation of COPD. The following lab work is done this morning: complete blood cell count, arterial blood gases, and an electrolyte panel consisting of K^+, Na^+, Cl^-, carbon dioxide, blood urea nitrogen, and fasting blood glucose. Which laboratory data will require immediate follow-up?
   (a.) PaO_2 WNL
   b. Increased RBCs
   c. Increased $PaCO_2$
   d. Hgb WNL

   Rationale: The answer is (a). Hypoxemia provides the stimulus for the respiratory drive in client with COPD. Increased oxygen levels may depress the respiratory drive. Options (b) and (c) are expected findings. Option (d) does not require immediate follow-up.

3. The client is admitted with an acute exacerbation of COPD. Which assessment finding is most indicative of a potential complication?
   (a.) R 32, increasingly anxious and restless
   b. Using accessory muscles during respiration
   c. Pulse oximetry 92%, pursed-lip breathing
   d. Expectorating copious amount of white phlegm

   Rationale: The answer is (a). Increasing anxiousness and restlessness are signs indicating hypoxemia. Options (b), (c), (d) are expected findings for a client with an exacerbation of COPD.

THE PATIENT WITH A CHEST TUBE

Mr. G, 23 years old, has been in the hospital for 2 days after being stabbed in the chest. He has a posterior chest tube connected to a Pleur-Evac system. You are assigned to his care and the nursing care Kardex contains the following information:

VS q4h I & O (✔) Amb with assist prn O_2 @ 2-3L/NP/Pulse ox q4h Chest tube to low con't suction	IV: D5/0.45 NS q12h IVPB cefazolin 1G IV q6h Chest x-ray today ABG today	Diet: Soft Routine med: Colace 100 mg po daily

The 7:00 AM report indicates that he had a restful night. Chest tube drainage was 15 mL. Midnight VS are T 99° F, P 90, R 22, BP 128/74. Pulse oximetry at 4:00 AM was 95%.

Instructions: Prioritize the five **nursing interventions** as you would do them to take care of Mr. G. Write a number in the box to identify the order of your interventions (#1 = first intervention, #2 = second intervention, etc.) and state a **rationale** for each intervention.

INTERVENTIONS	PRIORITY #	RATIONALE
• Check the pulse oximetry	☐	______
• Assess for fluctuation in the water-seal chamber and bubbling in the suction-control chamber	☐	______
• Check for the previous shift's fluid level marking on the tape	☐	______
• Assess chest tube patency and drainage	☐	______
• Ask Mr. G to cough and deep breathe	☐	______

KEY POINTS TO CONSIDER: ______

TWO

After breakfast, Mr. G is transported to the x-ray department by wheelchair. On his return to his room, you assess the following:

1. VS: T 99.8° F, P 92, R 26, BP 140/90
2. Complains of dyspnea, crackles auscultated, anxious
3. Oxygen off, oxygen saturation at 88%

Interactive activity: With a partner, **do the following:** (1) **select** the **one nursing diagnosis** that is of priority at this time, (2) **provide a rationale** for your selection, and (3) **list the nursing interventions** that assist you to meet the needs of the patient.

All of the following nursing diagnoses may apply to Mr. G:

Ineffective airway clearance, Ineffective breathing pattern, Impaired gas exchange, Risk for injury, Deficient knowledge, Fear, Anxiety, Risk for infection, Impaired tissue integrity

Nursing Diagnosis	Rationale	Nursing Interventions

One hour later, Mr. G becomes increasingly restless and, as you take his VS, he pulls out the chest tube.

Instructions: On the basis of the situation **1 hour later**, identify and write the **priority problem** in the box below. Then, starting with the small box labeled #1, **prioritize** the **nursing interventions** for this situation and **identify** your follow-up action plan for Mr. G.

NURSING INTERVENTIONS

A. Instruct Mr. G to take a deep breath and hold

B. Cover chest tube site with petrolatum gauze and 4 x 4 gauze

C. Apply gloves if possible

D. Increase oxygen to 3 L

E. Notify physician

F. Pinch chest tube site together

DECISION-MAKING DIAGRAM

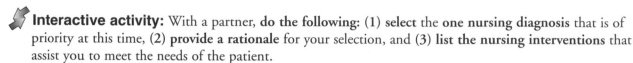

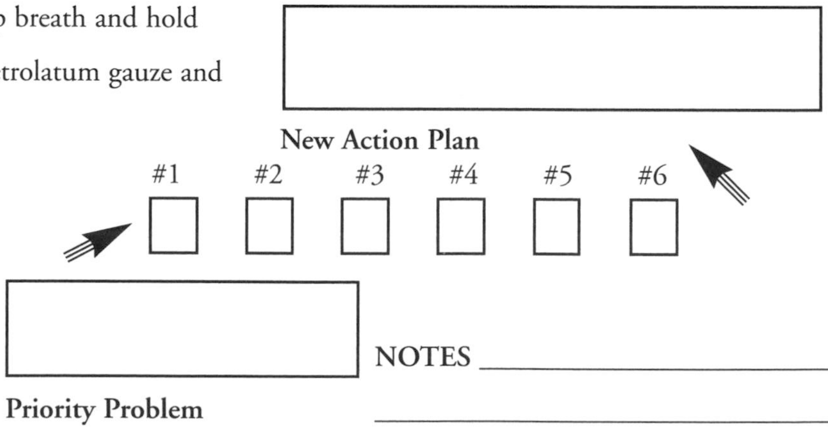

NOTES ____________________

____

APPLYING CRITICAL THINKING SKILLS TO TEST QUESTIONS

INSTRUCTIONS: Circle the one best answer for each test question. Write your rationale for selecting the answer. To enhance your learning and test-taking skills, discuss your answer and rationale with a partner. The answer and the rationale can be found on the back of this page.

TWO

1. The nurse is preparing to assist with the insertion of a chest tube that will be attached to a closed-chest drainage system without suction. In monitoring the closed-chest drainage system, the nurse would expect to initially assess for:
   a. fluctuation of water in the water-seal chamber during respirations.
   b. constant fluid fluctuations in the drainage-collection chamber.
   c. continuous bubbling in the suction-control chamber.
   d. occasional bubbling in the suction-control chamber.

   Rationale: ______________________________

2. The client has a chest tube connected to a closed-chest drainage system attached to suction and is being prepared to transfer to another room on a stretcher. To safely transport the client, it is most important for the nurse to:
   a. clamp the chest tube during the transport.
   b. get a portable suction before transferring the client.
   c. keep the closed-chest drainage system below the level of the chest.
   d. place the closed-chest drainage system next to the client on the stretcher.

   Rationale: ______________________________

3. The physician is preparing to remove the client's chest tube. Just before removing the chest tube, the physician tells the client to take a deep breath and hold it. The intervention is primarily done to:
   a. distract the client during the chest tube removal.
   b. minimize the negative pressure within the pleural space.
   c. decrease the degree of discomfort to the client.
   d. increase the intrathoracic pressure temporarily during removal.

   Rationale: ______________________________

ANSWER KEY FOR APPLYING CRITICAL THINKING SKILLS TO TEST QUESTIONS

HELPFUL HINTS: Read all test questions carefully. Identify key words in the question that will guide you in answering the question. In these test questions the **key words** to consider are **"initially,"** **"most important,"** and **"primarily."** Compare your rationale with the one in the test question.

1. The nurse is preparing to assist with the insertion of a chest tube that will be attached to a closed-chest drainage system without suction. In monitoring the closed-chest drainage system, the nurse would expect to initially assess for:
   (a.) fluctuation of water in the water-seal chamber during respirations.
   b. constant fluid fluctuations in the drainage-collection chamber.
   c. continuous bubbling in the suction-control chamber.
   d. occasional bubbling in the suction-control chamber.

   Rationale: The answer is (a). Fluctuations of water during inspiration and expiration in the water-seal chamber indicates normal functioning. Option (b) should not be seen in the collection chamber. Options (c) and (d) should not be seen because suction has not been applied to the suction-control chamber.

2. The client has a chest tube connected to a closed-chest drainage system attached to suction and is being prepared to transfer to another room on a stretcher. To safely transport the client, it is most important for the nurse to:
   a. clamp the chest tube during the transport.
   b. get a portable suction before transferring the client.
   (c.) keep the closed-chest drainage system below the level of the chest.
   d. place the closed-chest drainage system next to the client on the stretcher.

   Rationale: The answer is (c). Keeping the closed-chest drainage system below the level of the chest allows for continuous drainage and prevents any back flow pressure. Options (a) and (d) should not be done because they will increase pressure in the pleural space. Option (b) is not the most important.

3. The physician is preparing to remove the client's chest tube. Just before removing the chest tube, the physician tells the client to take a deep breath and hold it. The intervention is primarily done to:
   a. distract the client during the chest tube removal.
   b. minimize the negative pressure within the pleural space.
   c. decrease the degree of discomfort to the client.
   (d.) increase the intrathoracic pressure temporarily during removal.

   Rationale: The answer is (d). This is done to decrease the risk of atmospheric air entering the pleural space during removal. Options (a) and (c) are not the primary reasons for this intervention. Option (b) is not correct since negative pressure is desired within the lung.

THE PATIENT WITH UROSEPSIS

Mr. TD, 79 years old, was admitted today to the hospital with the diagnosis of urosepsis. He has an IV of D5/0.45 NS infusing at 100 mL/hr. Rocephin 1 g IVPB qAM is ordered. He is on I & O q8h, soft diet, bathroom privileges with assistance and Tylenol tabs ii po q4h for temperature >38° C. The day shift nurse indicated his VS were T 38° C, P 78, R 22, BP 146/88 at 2:00 PM. The nurse also said that he was more restless this afternoon and had been trying to get out of bed and seemed somewhat disoriented. He did not receive Tylenol but an order for a vest restraint was obtained and has been applied. You have been assigned as his nurse for the evening shift.

Instructions: Prioritize the following **nursing interventions** as you, the nurse, would do them to initially take care of Mr. TD. Write a number in the box to identify the order of your interventions (#1 = first intervention, #2 = second intervention, etc.) and state a **rationale** for each intervention.

INTERVENTIONS	PRIORITY #	RATIONALE
• Administer Tylenol tabs ii po if necessary	☐	______
• Take VS	☐	______
• Gather urinary output data	☐	______
• Check the vest restraint	☐	______
• Perform a body systems physical assessment	☐	______

KEY POINTS TO CONSIDER: ______

You perform a follow-up assessment at 7:00 PM and note the following:

1. VS: T 38.5° C, P 88, R 22, BP 120/76
2. Fine crackles audible on auscultation in the bilateral lower lung fields
3. He is sleepy
4. He was incontinent of a scant amount of urine

 Interactive activity: With a partner, **do the following:** (1) **select** the **one nursing diagnosis** that is of priority at this time, (2) **provide a rationale** for your selection, and (3) **list the nursing interventions** that assist to meet the needs of the patient.

All of the following nursing diagnoses may apply to Mr. TD:

> Risk for impaired skin integrity, Impaired urinary elimination, Risk for injury, Disturbed thought processes, Hyperthermia, Deficient fluid volume, Imbalanced nutrition: less than body requirements, Ineffective breathing pattern, Fatigue

Nursing Diagnosis	Rationale	Nursing Interventions

As you take his **8:00 PM** vital signs, you note the following signs and symptoms: Lethargic, skin very warm and flushed, VS: T 39.1° C, P 130, R 28, BP 90/54

Instructions: Based on the situation at **8:00 PM**, identify and write the **priority problem** in the box below. Then, starting with the small box labeled **#1**, **prioritize** the **nursing interventions** for this situation and **identify** your follow-up action plan for Mr. TD.

NURSING INTERVENTIONS

A. Check oxygen saturation level

B. Place in modified Trendelenburg position

C. Prepare to insert indwelling urinary catheter

D. Take vital signs

E. Document findings

F. Notify physician

DECISION-MAKING DIAGRAM

New Action Plan

#1 #2 #3 #4 #5 #6

☐ ☐ ☐ ☐ ☐ ☐

NOTES _____

Priority Problem _____

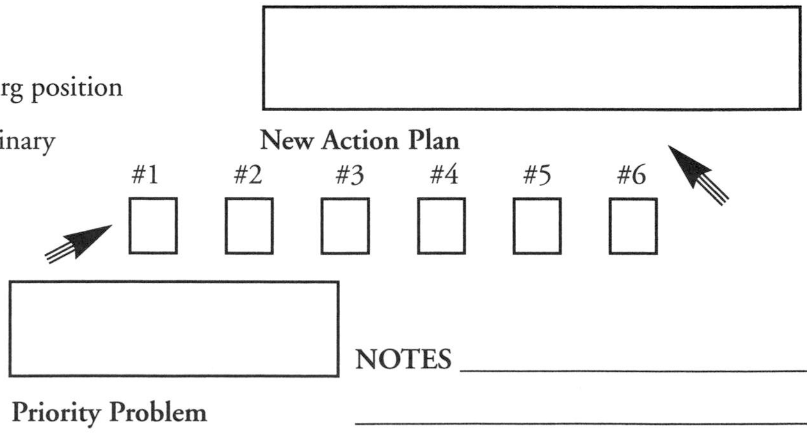

THE PATIENT WITH A TRANSURETHRAL RESECTION OF THE PROSTATE

Mr. J, 68 years old, had a TURP this morning after having been diagnosed with benign prostatic hypertrophy. The following postop orders have been noted:

VS q4h I & O - qs Antiembolic hose × 24 hr Sequential teds × 24 hr Up in chair this PM	IV: D5/045 NS @ 100 mL/hr IV site: RFA # 20 g 3-way urinary catheter to gravity with continuous irrigation of NS to keep UA free of clots	Diet: Clear liquids this PM PRN Medication: B&O supp. q4h prn bladder spasms

As you enter his room you notice that his urinary drainage bag is almost full and the normal saline irrigation bag is empty.

Instructions: Prioritize the five **nursing interventions** as you would do them to take care of Mr. J. Write a number in the box to identify the order of your interventions (#1 = first intervention, #2 = second intervention, etc.) and state a **rationale** for each intervention.

INTERVENTIONS	PRIORITY #	RATIONALE
• Take VS	☐	__________
• Assess continuous urinary irrigation system	☐	__________
• Empty urinary drainage bag	☐	__________
• Perform a body systems physical assessment	☐	__________
• Hang new normal saline solution irrigation bag	☐	__________

KEY POINTS TO CONSIDER: ____________________

On the first postop day you assess the following on Mr. J:

1. VS: T 99.6° F, P 88, R 20, BP 150/88
2. Urine pinkish, no clots
3. Grimaces and says, "I didn't think it would be this tough."
4. Urinary catheter taped to thigh

Interactive activity: With a partner, **do the following:** (1) **select** the **one nursing diagnosis** that is of priority at this time, (2) **provide a rationale** for your selection, and (3) **list the nursing interventions** that assist you to meet the needs of the patient.

All of the following nursing diagnoses may apply to Mr. J:

Risk for infection, Impaired tissue integrity, Excess fluid volume, Deficient knowledge, Anxiety, Risk for injury, Impaired urinary elimination, Pain, Ineffective sexuality patterns, Self-esteem: situational, low, Ineffective tissue perfusion

Nursing Diagnosis	Rationale	Nursing Interventions

The normal saline irrigation is discontinued at 12:00 noon the first postop day. Toward the end of the shift (**3:00 PM**), you **assess** the following on Mr. J: complaints of pain, no output since 12:00 PM, abdominal distention, and Mr. J is somewhat restless.

Instructions: On the basis of the **3:00 PM assessment**, identify and write the **priority problem** in the box below. Then, starting with the small box labeled **#1**, **prioritize** the **nursing interventions** for this situation and **identify** your follow-up action plan for Mr. J.

NURSING INTERVENTIONS

A. Take the vital signs

B. Inform MD

C. Prepare to do a urinary irrigation

D. Give an antispasmodic

E. Place in low- to semi-Fowler's position

F. Encourage fluids

DECISION-MAKING DIAGRAM

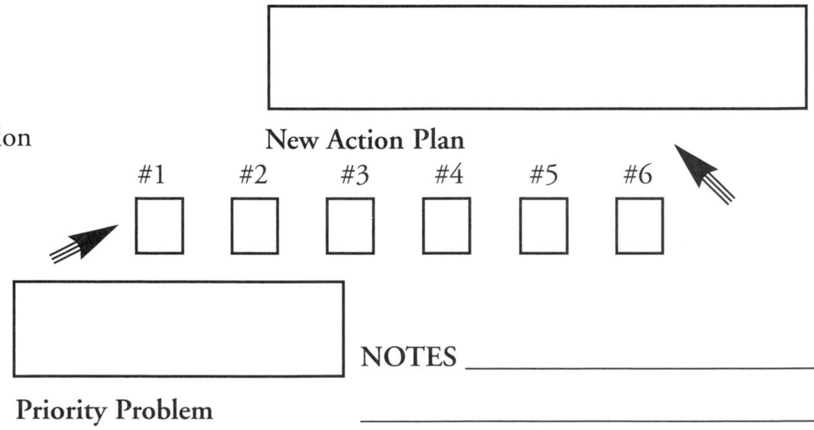

NOTES ____________________

____

TWO

APPLYING CRITICAL THINKING SKILLS TO TEST QUESTIONS

INSTRUCTIONS: Circle the one best answer for each test question. Write your rationale for selecting the answer. To enhance your learning and test-taking skills, discuss your answer and rationale with a partner. The answer and the rationale can be found on the back of this page.

1. The client is 1 day postop TURP. He has a three-way indwelling urinary catheter with continuous bladder irrigation. During change-of-shift report, the nurse learns that the client's output was 1700 mL. A priority nursing intervention is for the nurse to:
   a. check the client's oral and parenteral intake for the previous shift.
   b. know the amount of irrigation fluid that infused during the previous shift.
   c. assess if the client has passed any urinary clots through the catheter.
   d. ensure that the urinary output is yellow to pinkish in color.

   Rationale: ____________________

2. The physician orders continuous bladder irrigation for a client who had a TURP this morning. To effectively implement this order, it is most important for the nurse to infuse the irrigation solution:
   a. to maintain urine output clear to light pink in color.
   b. when the urine is red with visible clots.
   c. so that the intake equals the output.
   d. at a rate of 50 mL/hr.

   Rationale: ____________________

3. The client is 2 days postop TURP and is complaining of an increasing urge to void. The client has a three-way urinary catheter with continuous bladder irrigation. After assessment that the catheter is patent and is draining freely, the priority nursing intervention is to:
   a. reassure the client that the catheter is draining appropriately.
   b. document the client's complaints and assessment findings.
   c. give the client antispasmodic medication.
   d. notify the physician.

   Rationale: ____________________

ANSWER KEY FOR APPLYING CRITICAL THINKING SKILLS TO TEST QUESTIONS

HELPFUL HINTS: Read all test questions carefully. Identify key words in the question that will guide you in answering the question. In these test questions the **key words** to consider are "**priority**" and "**most important.**" Compare your rationale with the one in the test question.

1. The client is 1 day postop TURP. He has a three-way indwelling urinary catheter with continuous bladder irrigation. During change-of-shift report, the nurse learns that the client's output was 1700 mL. A priority nursing intervention is for the nurse to:
   a. check the client's oral and parenteral intake for the previous shift.
   (b.) know the amount of irrigation fluid that infused during the previous shift.
   c. assess if the client has passed any urinary clots through the catheter.
   d. ensure that the urinary output is yellow to pinkish in color.

   Rationale: The answer is (b). It is important to know the amount of irrigation solution that infused in order to assess the actual urinary output. Options (a), (c), and (d) are good interventions but not of priority.

2. The physician orders continuous bladder irrigation for a client who had a TURP this morning. To effectively implement this order, it is most important for the nurse to infuse the irrigation solution:
   (a.) to maintain urine output clear to light pink in color.
   b. when the urine is red with visible clots.
   c. so that the intake equals the output.
   d. at a rate of 50 mL/hr.

   Rationale: The answer is (a). Continuous irrigation is given to prevent clot formation and prevent obstruction of the catheter. Options (b), (c), and (d) are not appropriate interventions.

3. The client is 2 days postop TURP and is complaining of an increasing urge to void. The client has a three-way urinary catheter with continuous bladder irrigation. After assessment that the catheter is patent and is draining freely, the priority nursing intervention is to:
   a. reassure the client that the catheter is draining appropriately.
   b. document the client's complaints and assessment findings.
   (c.) give the client antispasmodic medication.
   d. notify the physician.

   Rationale: The answer is (c). Bladder spasms can cause the client to feel an urge to void. Options (a) and (b) do not address the client's current need. Option (d) is not appropriate at this time.

THE PATIENT RECEIVING A BLOOD TRANSFUSION

Mr. TA, 34 years old, was admitted after a motor vehicle accident: pedestrian versus car. He sustained multiple injuries throughout his body. He will receive 2 units of whole blood this morning. He has NS 0.9% infusing at TKO rate through a Y-type blood administration set, and he has a 19-gauge cannula in the RFA. The MD orders to infuse each unit over 3 to 4 hours. As you get out of the report, the lab notifies you that the first unit of blood is ready.

Instructions: Prioritize the five **nursing interventions** as you would do them to take care of Mr. TA. Write a number in the box to identify the order of your interventions (#1 = first intervention, #2 = second intervention, etc.) and state a **rationale** for each intervention.

INTERVENTIONS	PRIORITY #	RATIONALE
• Take an initial set of vital signs	☐	__________
• Pick up the blood from the lab	☐	__________
• Assess the IV site	☐	__________
• Start the transfusion	☐	__________
• Verify MD order, patient ID, and blood compatability	☐	__________

KEY POINTS TO CONSIDER: __________

TWO

You assess the following during the start of the transfusion on Mr. TA:

1. VS: T 97.6° F, P 80, R 18, BP 136/78 (pretransfusion)
2. VS: T 98.2° F, P 90, R 22, BP 130/70 (15 minutes after the start of the transfusion)
3. No complaints of itching
4. Transfusion rate increased to 100 mL/hr

Interactive activity: With a partner, **do the following:** (1) **select** the **one nursing diagnosis** that is of priority at this time, (2) **provide a rationale** for your selection, and (3) **list the nursing interventions** that assist to meet the needs of the patient.

All of the following nursing diagnoses may apply to Mr. TA:

Risk for infection, Fatigue, Risk for excess fluid volume, Deficient fluid volume, Deficient knowledge, Anxiety, Risk for injury, Pain

Nursing Diagnosis	Rationale	Nursing Interventions

After 20 minutes Mr. TA's **assessment** includes: Skin flushed, P 120, R 32, BP 100/60, complains of chest pain and chills

Instructions: Based on the above **assessment**, identify and write the **priority problem** in the box below. Then, starting with the small box labeled **#1**, **prioritize** the **nursing interventions** for this situation and **identify** your follow-up action plan for Mr. TA.

NURSING INTERVENTIONS

A. Stop the transfusion

B. Inform MD

C. Save the next voided specimen

D. Start 0.9% NS at TKO rate

E. Take VS

F. Save the transfusion unit

DECISION-MAKING DIAGRAM

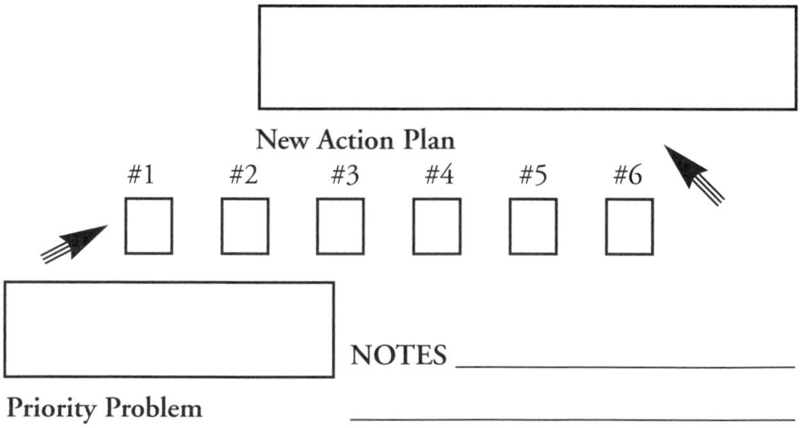

THE PATIENT WITH NEUTROPENIA

Mrs. K, 50 years old, was admitted 2 days ago with neutropenia. Her current white blood cell count is 750/mm^3. During morning report you note the following from the nursing care Kardex:

VS q4 I & O Neutropenic precautions (✓) Bone marrow biopsy—today CBC with diff—today Chest x-ray done	Diet: ↑ protein, ↑ calorie (no raw vegetables/fresh fruit) IV: D_5W @ 125 mL/hr IV site: RFA (inserted 2 days ago)	Routine medication: Colace 100 mg po daily 0900 PRN medication: Tylenol 325 tabs ii q4h po prn Temp greater than 100.4° F

Instructions: Prioritize the five **nursing interventions** as you would do them to take care of Mrs. K. Write a number in the box to identify the order of your interventions (#1 = first intervention, #2 = second intervention, etc.) and state a **rationale** for each intervention.

INTERVENTIONS	PRIORITY #	RATIONALE
• Wash hands	☐	______________
• Assess the IV site	☐	______________
• Provide fresh water at bedside	☐	______________
• Assess oral mucosa	☐	______________
• Take the vital signs	☐	______________

KEY POINTS TO CONSIDER: ______________________________

TWO

Mrs. K is diagnosed with acute leukemia. Your follow-up assessment includes:

1. Hgb 9.8 g/dL, hematocrit 29%
2. White blood cell count 900/mm^3
3. Using antifungal medication as ordered
4. Platelet count 100,000/mm^3

Interactive activity: With a partner, **do the following:** (1) **select** the **one nursing diagnosis** that is of priority at this time, (2) **provide a rationale** for your selection, and (3) **list the nursing interventions** that assist to meet the needs of the patient.

All of the following nursing diagnoses may apply to Mrs. K:

Risk for infection, Fatigue, Imbalanced nutrition: less than body requirements, Deficient knowledge, Anxiety, Risk for injury, Impaired oral mucous membrane, Activity intolerance, Risk for impaired skin integrity, Social isolation, Ineffective tissue perfusion

Nursing Diagnosis	Rationale	Nursing Interventions

The following day, Mrs. K's **assessment findings** are significant for: platelet count 30,000/mm^3; bleeding time prolonged, oral petechiae, hemoptysis, tachypnea, dyspnea, and a current nosebleed.

Instructions: On the basis of the above **assessment**, identify and write the **priority problem** in the box below. Then, starting with the small box labeled #1, **prioritize** the **nursing interventions** for this situation and **identify** your follow-up action plan for Mrs. K.

NURSING INTERVENTIONS

A. Take the vital signs

B. Assess other site for signs and symptoms of bleeding

C. Assess neurologic status

D. Place in high-Fowler's position

E. Apply direct pressure to nose

F. Inform physician

DECISION-MAKING DIAGRAM

New Action Plan

#1 #2 #3 #4 #5 #6

Priority Problem

NOTES ______________________

____

THE PATIENT WITH A HIP FRACTURE

Mrs. T, 72 years old, fell at home and was admitted to the hospital with a fracture of the right hip. She was alert and oriented on admission. After the initial workup, she was taken to surgery for an open reduction with internal fixation (ORIF) of her right hip. On her first postop day, her right hip dressing has a small amount of dried, dark red drainage. She has an IV of D_5/0.45 NS at 75 mL/hr, oxygen at 2 L/nasal cannula, clear liquid diet, and circulation, movement, sensation, and temperature (CMST) neurovascular checks q4h to the right leg for the first 24 hours. The following medications are ordered: PCA with morphine sulfate delivering 1 mg/hr continuously, $FeSO_4$ 325 mg po tid with meals (start when on regular diet), Colace 100 mg po daily. She is very restless and confused this morning.

Instructions: Prioritize the five interventions according to Mrs. T's current needs. Write a number in the box to identify the order of your interventions (#1 = first intervention, #2 = second intervention, etc.) and state a **rationale** for each intervention.

INTERVENTIONS	PRIORITY #	RATIONALE
• Assess surgical dressing	☐	
• Take VS	☐	
• Assess pain level	☐	
• Check oxygen saturation level	☐	
• Check neurovascular status of right leg (CMST)	☐	

KEY POINTS TO CONSIDER:

TWO

During the follow-up assessment for the **first postop day**, you note the following:

1. Pedal pulse present; weak in the right foot, stronger on left foot
2. Hemoglobin 10.5 g/dL and hematocrit 32%
3. Bowel sounds hypoactive in all quadrants
4. Crackles in the lower bases of the lung

Interactive activity: With a partner, **do the following:** (1) **select** the **one nursing diagnosis** that is of priority at this time, (2) **provide a rationale** for your selection, and (3) **list the nursing interventions** that assist to meet the needs of the patient.

All of the following nursing diagnoses may apply to Mrs. T:

Acute pain, Risk for infection, Risk for impaired skin integrity, Impaired urinary elimination, Impaired gas exchange, Fatigue, Impaired physical mobility, Ineffective tissue perfusion

Nursing Diagnosis	Rationale	Nursing Interventions

On the second postop day Mrs. T is still very confused and is trying to get out of bed. She has bilateral scattered crackles in the lungs, shortness of breath on exertion, R 32, and a nonproductive cough.

Instructions: Based on the situation above, identify and write the **priority problem** in the box below. Then, starting with the small box labeled **#1**, **prioritize** the **nursing interventions** for this situation and **identify** your plan for follow-up care for Mrs. T.

NURSING INTERVENTIONS

A. Take VS

B. Check oxygen saturation

C. Stay with patient

D. Encourage incentive spirometer hourly

E. Call physician

F. Encourage fluids

DECISION-MAKING DIAGRAM

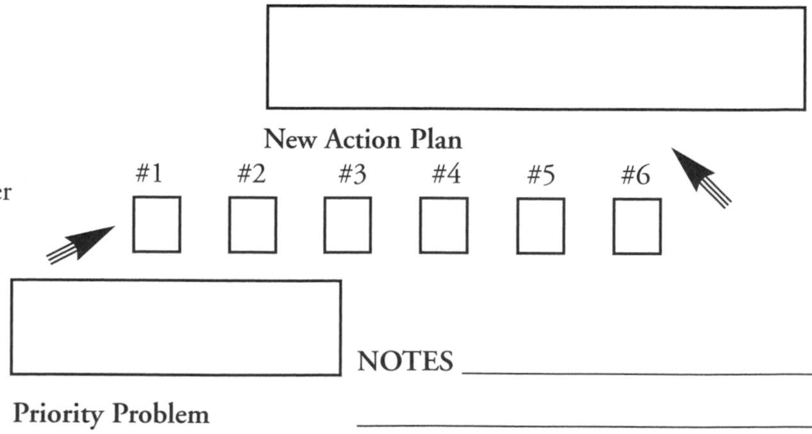

NOTES ______________________

____

APPLYING CRITICAL THINKING SKILLS TO TEST QUESTIONS

INSTRUCTIONS: Circle the one best answer for each test question. Write your rationale for selecting the answer. To enhance your learning and test-taking skills, discuss your answer and rationale with a partner. The answer and the rationale can be found on the back of this page.

1. The nurse is caring for an 82-year-old client who is 1 day postop left hip replacement. The client has a primary IV infusing at 100 mL/hr, a patient-controlled analgesic device, and a urinary catheter. After assessing the client, the nurse determines that the client is pleasant and cooperative but forgetful. In the afternoon, the nurse notes that the client has become increasingly restless. It is most important for the nurse to:
   a. apply soft restraints.
   b. notify the physician.
   c. check the patient-controlled analgesic device.
   d. assess the client's medical history for dementia.

   Rationale: ____

2. The nurse is delegating the care of a 79-year-old client 2 days postop hip replacement to a nursing assistant who routinely works on a postpartum unit. Which instruction given to the nursing assistant is of priority initially?
   a. Have the client cough and deep breathe q2h.
   b. Total the intake and output at 1400.
   c. Use a fracture bedpan on the client.
   d. Wash the client's skin with a mild soap.

   Rationale: ____

3. The nurse is assisting a client to get out of a chair after having a right hip replacement 3 days ago. The client suddenly complains of pain and tells the nurse that it hurts too much to walk. Which nursing intervention is of priority?
   a. Encourage the client to put most of the weight on the left leg.
   b. Support the client's right side as the client is asked to stand up.
   c. Assess the client's right hip and leg.
   d. Administer pain medication.

   Rationale: ____

ANSWER KEY FOR APPLYING CRITICAL THINKING SKILLS TO TEST QUESTIONS

HELPFUL HINTS: Read all test questions carefully. Identify key words in the question that will guide you in answering the question. In these test questions the **key words** to consider are **"most important," "priority initially,"** and **"priority."** Compare your rationale with the one in the test question.

1. The nurse is caring for an 82-year-old client who is 1 day postop left hip replacement. The client has a primary IV infusing at 100 mL/hr, a patient-controlled analgesic device, and a urinary catheter. After assessing the client, the nurse determines that the client is pleasant and cooperative but forgetful. In the afternoon, the nurse notes that the client has become increasingly restless. It is most important for the nurse to:
   a. apply soft restraints.
   b. notify the physician.
   c. check the patient-controlled analgesic device.
   d. assess the client's medical history for dementia.

   Rationale: The answer is (c). Pain may be a contributing factor to the client's restlessness. The patient-controlled analgesic device should be checked to see whether the client has used it to control the pain. Options (a), (b), and (d) are not appropriate interventions.

2. The nurse is delegating the care of a 79-year-old client 2 days postop hip replacement to a nursing assistant who routinely works on a postpartum unit. Which instruction given to the nursing assistant is of priority initially?
   a. Have the client cough and deep breathe q2h.
   b. Total the intake and output at 1400.
   c. Use a fracture bedpan on the client.
   d. Wash the client's skin with a mild soap.

   Rationale: The answer is (c). A fracture bedpan will minimize putting stress on the hip area and preventing hip dislocation. Options (a), (b), and (d) are important, but instructing a new nursing assistant on how to prevent complications is of priority.

3. The nurse is assisting a client to get out of a chair after having a right hip replacement 3 days ago. The client suddenly complains of pain and tells the nurse that it hurts too much to walk. Which nursing intervention is of priority?
   a. Encourage the client to put most of the weight on the left leg.
   b. Support the client's right side as the client is asked to stand up.
   c. Assess the client's right hip and leg.
   d. Administer pain medication.

   Rationale: The answer is (c). Increased pain may indicate hip dislocation. Options (a), (b), and (d) are good interventions, but the nurse should assess the surgical site before continuing with any other intervention.

THE PATIENT WITH A FRACTURED TIBIA

Mr. W, 26 years old, was admitted with a left fractured tibia. He was taken to surgery and is now being transferred to the orthopedic unit. He has a long leg cast on the left leg. His postop orders are transcribed to the nursing care Kardex:

VS q4h I & O (✓) Neurovascular cks (circ. movement, sensation, temp) q4h Elevate left leg on (1) pillow	1 L D_5W q10h—discontinue when taking fluids well Teach crutch walking in AM by physical therapy	Diet: Clear liquids → Reg. Medications PCA—Dilaudid 0.2 mg/hr

You are assigned to Mr. W as he is taken into his room. You note that he is alert, the left leg cast is damp and clean, and an IV is infusing into his right hand.

Instructions: Prioritize the five **nursing interventions** as you would do them to take care of Mr. W. Write a number in the box to identify the order of your interventions (#1 = first intervention, #2 = second intervention, etc.) and state a **rationale** for each intervention.

INTERVENTIONS	PRIORITY #	RATIONALE
• Take VS	☐	______
• Neurovascular assessment of both extremities	☐	______
• Assess cast for dryness, signs of drainage, and sharp edges	☐	______
• Use palms of hands to elevate cast on a pillow	☐	______
• Teach isometric exercises	☐	______

KEY POINTS TO CONSIDER: ______

TWO

On the morning of the first postop day, you note the following:

1. Mr. W is requesting pain medication q4h
2. Left pedal pulses present, edema 2+
3. Capillary refill >2 seconds, moves left toes
4. Mr. W is taking fluids and voiding sufficient quantity
5. MD orders CPK, LDH, and SGOT

Interactive activity: With a partner, **do the following:** (1) **select** the **one nursing diagnosis** that is of priority at this time, (2) **provide a rationale** for your selection, and (3) **list the nursing interventions** that assist you to meet the needs of the patient.

All of the following nursing diagnoses may apply to Mr. W:

Risk for injury, Deficient knowledge, Risk for infection, Risk for impaired skin integrity, Impaired physical mobility, Fear, Ineffective tissue perfusion, Pain, Activity intolerance, Impaired tissue integrity, Anxiety, Risk for peripheral neurovascular dysfunction

Nursing Diagnosis	Rationale	Nursing Interventions

Mr. W refuses lunch and you assess: complaints of increased pain, especially with elevation of the leg; numbness and tingling; left pedal pulse weak, cool

Instructions: On the basis of this new information, identify and write the **priority problem** in the box below. Then, starting with the small box labeled #1, **prioritize** the **nursing interventions** for this situation and **identify** your follow-up action plan for Mr. W.

NURSING INTERVENTIONS

A. Inform MD stat

B. Prepare to have cast bivalved

C. Ensure left extremity is at heart level

D. Monitor left pedal pulse

E. Take VS

F. Stay with patient

DECISION-MAKING DIAGRAM

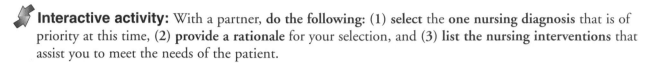

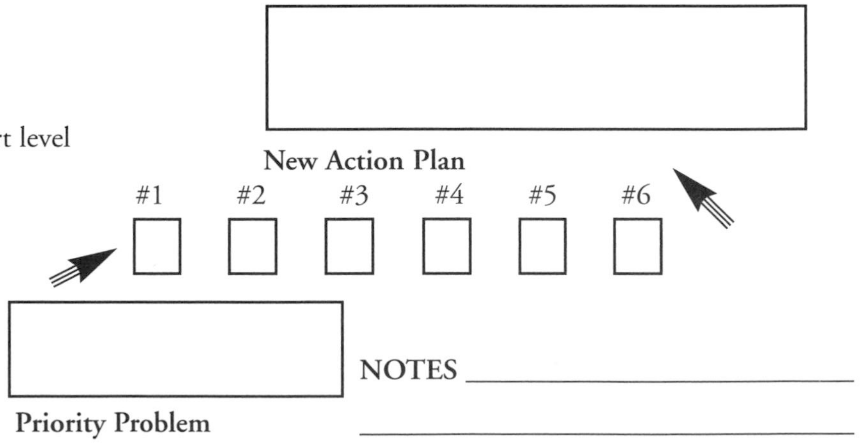

THE PATIENT WITH CATARACT SURGERY

Mrs. G, 72 years old, has senile cataracts and has been instilling mydriatic eye drops. Her vision has progressively worsened and she is scheduled today for a right cataract extraction in the outpatient clinic. The MD orders the following preop preparation: NPO; instill mydriatic and cycloplegic eye drops 1 hour before surgery; Valium 5 mg po 1 hour before surgery. Mrs. G arrives at the outpatient clinic at 0800 and she is scheduled for surgery at 1000.

Instructions: Prioritize the five **nursing interventions** as you would do them to take care of Mrs. G. Write a number in the box to identify the order of your interventions (#1 = first intervention, #2 = second intervention, etc.) and state a **rationale** for each intervention.

TWO

INTERVENTIONS	PRIORITY #	RATIONALE
• Provide information regarding preop preparation	☐	______
• Begin to instill ordered eye drops	☐	______
• Have patient void	☐	______
• Take VS	☐	______
• Ensure the surgical consent is signed before initiating preop preparation	☐	______

KEY POINTS TO CONSIDER: ______

Mrs. G had an intraocular lens implant and is taken to the recovery room. She has an eye patch on her right eye, and you assess the following:

1. No complaints of pain, P 88, BP 130/82
2. Eye patch clean and dry
3. Readily responds to verbal stimuli

 Interactive activity: With a partner, **do the following:** (1) **select** the **one nursing diagnosis** that is of priority at this time, (2) **provide a rationale** for your selection, and (3) **list the nursing interventions** that assist to meet the needs of the patient.

All of the following nursing diagnoses may apply to Mrs. G:

Risk for injury, Deficient knowledge, Disturbed sensory perception, Fear, Anxiety, Risk for self-care deficit, Risk for infection, Ineffective health maintenance, Impaired home maintenance, Sensory-perceptual alterations: visual

Nursing Diagnosis	Rationale	Nursing Interventions

One hour **postop** you assess Mrs. G and note the following: complaints of right brow pain, anxious, P 110, BP 128/80, coughing, and complaints of nausea

Instructions: Based on the **postop** assessment, identify and write the **priority problem** in the box below. Then, starting with the small box labeled **#1**, **prioritize** the **nursing interventions** for this situation and **identify** your follow-up action plan for Mrs. G.

NURSING INTERVENTIONS

A. Avoid rapid head movement

B. Administered antiemetic if ordered

C. Document findings/nursing care

D. Notify MD

E. Recheck pulse and BP

F. Stay with Mrs. G

DECISION-MAKING DIAGRAM

New Action Plan

#1 #2 #3 #4 #5 #6
☐ ☐ ☐ ☐ ☐ ☐

Priority Problem

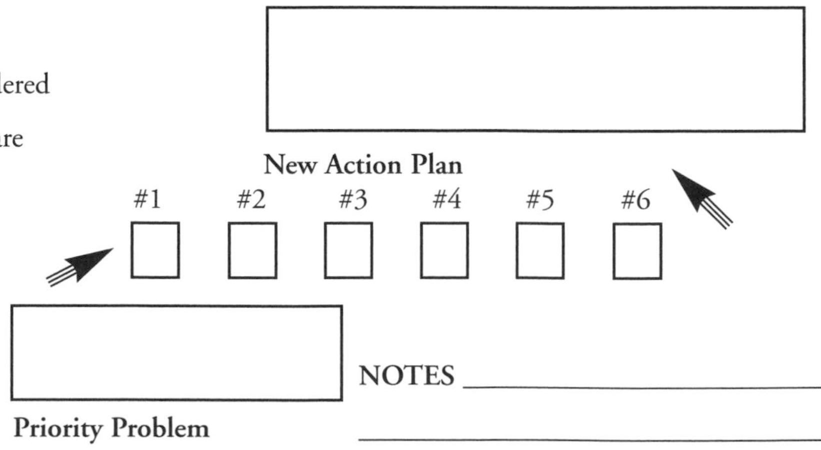

NOTES _____

THE PATIENT WITH A SEIZURE DISORDER

Mr. M, 20 years old, fell at home and was brought to the emergency department after it was noticed that he had lost consciousness for a few seconds. In the emergency department he indicated that he did not remember falling. His family history is significant for seizure disorders. Diagnostic studies were ordered and included an electroencephalogram, magnetic resonance imaging, serum blood glucose, complete blood cell count, blood urea nitrogen, and urinalysis drug screening. He was just transferred to the neurology unit from the emergency department. The current MD orders include seizure precautions, bed rest, soft diet, saline lock, VS, and neurologic checks q4h.

Instructions: Prioritize the following **nursing interventions** as you would do them to initially take care of Mr. M. Write a number in the box to identify the order of your interventions (#1 = first intervention, #2 = second intervention, etc.) and state a **rationale** for each intervention.

INTERVENTIONS	PRIORITY #	RATIONALE
• Orient Mr. M to his room	☐	___
• Assess neurologic status	☐	___
• Implement seizure precautions	☐	___
• Obtain admitting history	☐	___
• Inform of pertinent MD orders	☐	___

KEY POINTS TO CONSIDER: ___

Mr. M is diagnosed with a seizure disorder and is started on Depakote. In speaking with Mr. M, you gather the following:

1. Mr. M says that he has had similar episodes but never told anyone.
2. He remembers seeing "spots" before the episode.
3. No one in his family talked much about the relative who had seizures.

 Interactive activity: With a partner, **do the following:** (1) **select** the **one nursing diagnosis** that is of priority at this time, (2) **provide a rationale** for your selection, and (3) **list the nursing interventions** that assist you to meet the needs of the patient.

All of the following nursing diagnoses may apply to Mr. M:

Ineffective coping, Ineffective airway clearance, Risk for injury, Deficient knowledge, Disturbed self-concept, Social isolation, Fear, Anxiety, Disturbed thought processes, Risk for aspiration

Nursing Diagnosis	Rationale	Nursing Interventions

Several hours after admission, you hear a "cry" coming from Mr. M's room. You assess the following as you walk into the room: Tonic-clonic movements of the body, loss of consciousness, excessive salivation, some cyanosis, urinary incontinence, teeth clenched with cessation of tonic-clonic movements after 3 minutes.

Instructions: On the basis of the situation above, identify and write the **priority problem** in the box below. Then, starting with the small box labeled **#1**, **prioritize** the **nursing interventions** for this situation and identify your follow-up action plan for Mr. M.

NURSING INTERVENTIONS

A. Maintain a quiet environment

B. Assess for injury

C. Check airway patency

D. Document findings

E. Turn to side

F. Reorient patient

DECISION-MAKING DIAGRAM

New Action Plan

#1 #2 #3 #4 #5 #6

☐ ☐ ☐ ☐ ☐ ☐

Priority Problem

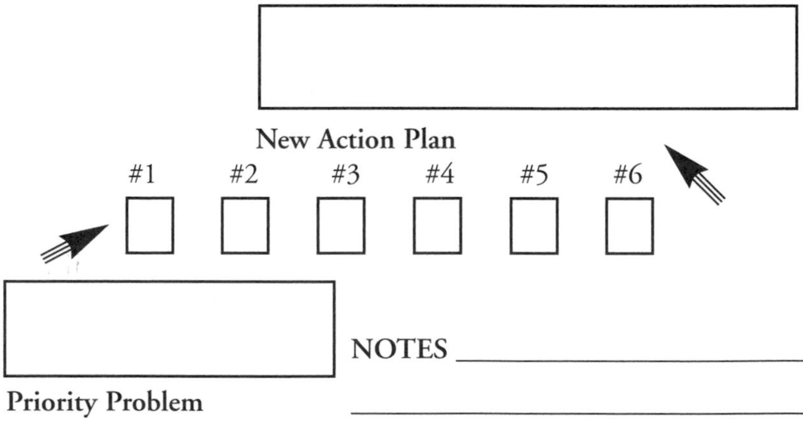

NOTES _____

APPLYING CRITICAL THINKING SKILLS TO TEST QUESTIONS

INSTRUCTIONS: Circle the one best answer for each test question. Write your rationale for selecting the answer. To enhance your learning and test-taking skills, discuss your answer and rationale with a partner. The answer and the rationale can be found on the back of this page.

1. The nurse documents the following after observing a client have a tonic-clonic seizure: "0930 Found client having jerky, involuntary movements of upper and lower extremities lasting 2 minutes, frothy saliva oozing from mouth, incontinent of urine." Which statement best describes the nurse's charting? The charting:
   a. is appropriate and describes the observations seen.
   b. should include the client's response and nursing interventions.
   c. should just indicate that the client had a tonic-clonic seizure.
   d. is lacking whether the client had an aura experience before the seizure.

   Rationale: ____

2. The nurse admits a client who is having uncontrolled generalized tonic-clonic seizures. In planning for potential complications, which nursing intervention is of priority?
   a. Have a tongue blade next to the client's bed.
   b. Have suction equipment available.
   c. Maintain side rails up at all times.
   d. Maintain a quiet environment.

   Rationale: ____

3. The nurse is caring for a client who is on phenytoin (Dilantin) 200 mg po tid and phenobarbital 20 mg po tid. Which assessment finding is most indicative of a common side effect of these medications?
   a. Gums red and swollen
   b. Complaints of constipation
   c. Respiratory depression
   d. Skin rash

   Rationale: ____

ANSWER KEY FOR APPLYING CRITICAL THINKING SKILLS TO TEST QUESTIONS

HELPFUL HINTS: Read all test questions carefully. Identify key words in the question that will guide you in answering the question. In these test questions the **key words** to consider are **"best,"** **"priority,"** and **"most indicative."** Compare your rationale with the one in the test question.

1. The nurse documents the following after observing a client have a tonic-clonic seizure: "0930 Found client having jerky, involuntary movements of upper and lower extremities lasting 2 minutes, frothy saliva oozing from mouth, incontinent of urine." Which statement best describes the nurse's charting? The charting:
   a. is appropriate and describes the observations seen.
   (b.) should include the client's response and nursing interventions.
   c. should just indicate that the client had a tonic-clonic seizure.
   d. is lacking whether the client had an aura experience before the seizure.

   Rationale: The answer is (b). Charting should include what is observed, the nursing interventions, and the client's response/reaction. Options (a), (c), and (d) do not include all the components necessary for legal documentation.

2. The nurse admits a client who is having uncontrolled generalized tonic-clonic seizures. In planning for potential complications, which nursing intervention is of priority?
   a. Have a tongue blade next to the client's bed.
   (b.) Have suction equipment available.
   c. Maintain side rails up at all times.
   d. Maintain a quiet environment.

   Rationale: The answer is (b). Suction equipment is necessary to clear oral secretions after the seizure and prevent aspiration. Options (c) and (d) are important, but preventing aspiration is of priority. Option (a) is not a current intervention.

3. The nurse is caring for a client who is on phenytoin (Dilantin) 200 mg po tid and phenobarbital 20 mg po tid. Which assessment finding is most indicative of a common side effect of these medications?
   (a.) Gums red and swollen
   b. Complaints of constipation
   c. Respiratory depression
   d. Skin rash

   Rationale: The answer is (a). Gingival hyperplasia is a common side effect seen with the administration of phenytoin. Meticulous oral hygiene is an important intervention. Option (b) is not a common side effect. Option (c) is a toxic reaction to phenobarbital, and option (d) is a toxic reaction to phenytoin.

THE PATIENT WITH A DO-NOT-RESUSCITATE ORDER

Mr. B, 83 years old, has terminal esophageal cancer. The following pertinent information is found in the nursing care rand:

Activity: Bed rest Vital signs: q4h O_2 sats: q4h Lives with son Hospital Day: #4	PEG tube insertion: 3 days ago Formula full strength: 50 mL/hr Ck residual q4h; if greater than 100 mL, hold feeding for 1 hour Morphine sulfate 2 mg IV q2h prn pain	IV: D_5/0.45 NS q12h Urinary catheter inserted on admission I & O q8h Code Status: No code

The 7:00 AM report indicates that his current respirations are 10 and he last received morphine sulfate at 6:00 AM. Residual urine at that time was 125 mL; tube feeding was stopped. IV has 200 mL left.

Instructions: Prioritize the five **nursing interventions** as you would do them to initially take care of Mr. B. Write a number in the box to identify the order of your interventions (#1= first intervention, #2 = second intervention, etc.) and state a **rationale** for each intervention.

INTERVENTIONS	PRIORITY #	RATIONALE
• Assess PEG tube residual	☐	______
• Take VS	☐	______
• Assess IV site and IV fluid level	☐	______
• Perform a body system assessment	☐	______
• Assess oxygen saturation level	☐	______

KEY POINTS TO CONSIDER: ______

At 11:00 AM Mr. B manifested the following signs and symptoms:

1. VS: P 76, R14, BP 118/64
2. Responds appropriately but is weak and lethargic
3. Urine is dark yellow; output 125 mL since 7:00 AM
4. Shortness of breath when turning; irregular breathing pattern

Interactive activity: With a partner, **do the following:** (1) **select** the **one nursing diagnosis** that is of priority at this time, (2) **provide a rationale** for your selection, and (3) **list the nursing interventions** that assist to meet the needs of the patient.

All of the following nursing diagnoses may apply to Mr. B:

Risk for infection, Pain, Anxiety, Impaired gas exchange, Imbalanced nutrition: less than body requirements, Risk for deficient fluid volume, Risk for impaired skin integrity, Ineffective tissue perfusion, Activity intolerance, Powerlessness, Social isolation

Nursing Diagnosis	Rationale	Nursing Interventions

At **2:00 PM** Mr. B is unresponsive to verbal stimuli. You assessed: VS: P 36, R 9, BP 80/50. Urine output unchanged since 11:00 AM. Lower extremities cool with cyanosis.

Instructions: Based on the **2:00 PM** assessment, identify and write the **priority problem** in the box below. Then, starting with the small box labeled **#1**, **prioritize** the **nursing interventions** for this situation and **identify** your plan for follow-up care for Mr. B.

NURSING INTERVENTIONS

A. Monitor VS

B. Check NCP for religious/cultural requests

C. Report findings to physician

D. Notify relatives

E. Provide comfort measures

F. Document findings

DECISION-MAKING DIAGRAM

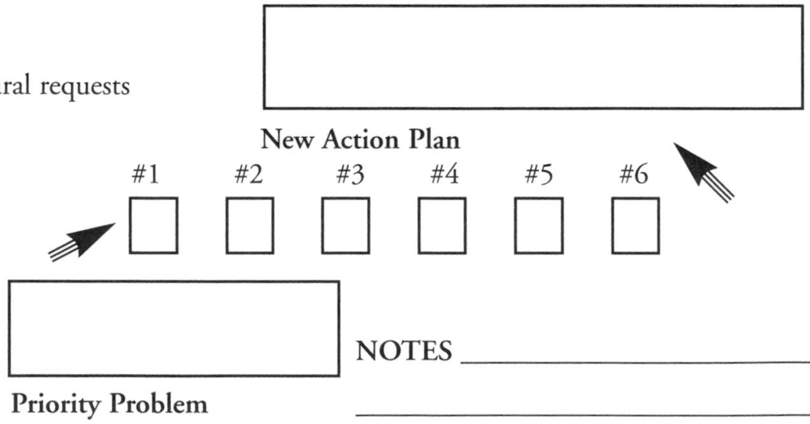

NOTES ______________________

____

LEGAL CONSIDERATIONS

Mrs. L is 1 day postop total abdominal hysterectomy. She is 42 years old. Meperidine 75 mg is ordered IM q3h prn for pain. She is on a clear liquid diet and has not voided since the urinary catheter was removed at noon. She is ambulating with assistance to the bathroom. The abdominal dressing is stained with dried dark red drainage. VS at noon are T 99° F, P 82, R 22, BP 130/76. Fine crackles are audible in the lower bases of the lung fields. It is 4:00 PM, and she is requesting pain medication. She states her pain level is 4. Her last pain shot was administered at 2:00 PM. An incentive spirometer is at the bedside.

Instructions: Prioritize the following **nursing interventions** as you, the nurse, would do them to initially take care of Mrs. L. Write a number in the box to identify the order of your interventions (#1 = first intervention, #2 = second intervention, etc.) and state a **rationale** for each intervention.

INTERVENTIONS	PRIORITY #	RATIONALE
• Inform Mrs. L that the pain medication is not due for another hour	☐	______
• Encourage coughing and deep breathing; demonstrate abdominal splinting; have patient use incentive spirometer q1h	☐	______
• Assist patient to ambulate to the bathroom	☐	______
• Take VS	☐	______
• Assess abdomen and surgical dressing	☐	______

KEY POINTS TO CONSIDER: ______

TWO

Mrs. L voids 400 mL after ambulating to the bathroom and states that she feels much better. She relates the following to you:

1. Her mother had a hysterectomy but died 10 days later from surgical complications.
2. She is glad that she does not have to worry about irregular periods any more.
3. She fully trusts her doctor but wonders whether the right thing was done.
4. She lives alone.

Interactive activity: With a partner, **do the following:** (1) **select** the **one nursing diagnosis** that is of priority at this time, (2) **provide a rationale** for your selection, and (3) **list the nursing interventions** that assist to meet the needs of the patient.

All of the following nursing diagnoses may apply to Mrs. L:

Risk for infection, Pain, Anxiety, Ineffective breathing pattern, Imbalanced nutrition: less than body requirements, Disturbed body image, Sexual dysfunction, Impaired skin integrity, Risk for activity intolerance, Deficient knowledge

Nursing Diagnosis	Rationale	Nursing Interventions

At 6:00 PM Mrs. L states that she is having pain. In fact, on a scale from 0-10, Mrs. L's pain is an 8. She has not received any pain medication since 2:00 PM. You take out an ampule labeled meperidine 100 mg/mL and administer 1 mL. Mrs. L asks whether the 75 mg of meperidine would help her since it did not help her before.

Instructions: Based on the situation above, identify and write the **priority problem** in the box below. Then, starting with the small box labeled **#1**, **prioritize** the **nursing interventions** for this situation and **identify** your follow-up action plan for Mrs. L.

NURSING INTERVENTIONS

A. Tell the patient you administered 100 mg of meperidine
B. Document drug and amount given
C. Monitor VS
D. Fill out an incident report
E. Notify your instructor
F. Notify physician

DECISION-MAKING DIAGRAM

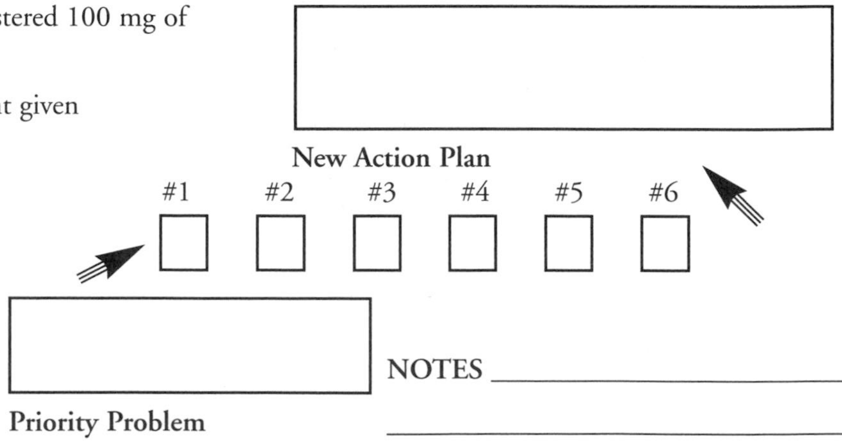

NOTES ______________________

____

Section Three - Applying the Critical Thinking Model

CLINICAL SITUATION #1

Intershift report at 0700:

"Mr. A, 72 years old, is 2 days postop small bowel resection. His NG tube is connected to low wall suction and is draining dark brown fluid. Vital signs at 0600: T 99.6° F, P 90, R 28, BP 160/94. IV D5/0.45 NS with 20 mEq KCl infusing at 125 mL into the right forearm. He is using the PCA machine. He slept most of the night and is now sitting in a chair. SOB was noted when he was transferred to the chair. There is 300 mL left in the IV."

Mr. A's current **flow charts** contain the following information:

Medication Record

Routine	Time Due
Lanoxin 0.25 mg IV daily	0900
Lasix 20 mg IVP daily	0900
Timolol 0.25% gtt i both eyes BID	1000
Protonix 40 mg IVPB daily	1000
Gentamicin 80 mg IVPB q8h	1400

PRN

Phenergan 25 mg IV/IM q4h N/V

PCA (morphine sulfate - 1 mg/hr continuous, 4-hour limit 30 mg)

Intake and Output Record

Night Shift @ 0600

Intake		Output	
PO =	0	UA void =	0
		Foley =	200
IV =	1000	N/G =	600
IVPB =	100		

Interactive activity: With a partner, **use the case study and the flow charts** to:

1. Identify the pertinent patient information made known to you in the *report.*	2. Identify the pertinent patient information made known to you in the *flow charts.*	3. Review the data in columns 1 and 2 and identify information that needs follow-up.

THREE

It is 0730 as you leave the report room. **Prioritize** your plan of care for the morning:

Time	Plan of Nursing Care

1200 nursing assessment: Oriented ×3, skin WNL, capillary refill <3 sec, turgor good, mucous membranes moist, pinkish, T. 99° F, P 88 and slightly irregular, R 24, BP 164/94. NG draining brownish fluid 100 mL since 0800. Bowel sounds present ×4, abd. soft. Foley catheter draining clear yellow urine.

Mr. A has minimal complaints and is visited by the physician at 1200. The physician leaves the following orders:

Remove Foley catheter now
Enc. incentive spirometer q1h ×10
Discontinue NG tube
DC Lasix
Lanoxin 0.25 mg po daily
Hgb & Hct today
Clear liquid diet

1. Identify the nursing interventions that require immediate follow-up.	2. Identify the nursing actions that you can delegate/assign to unlicensed personnel.

For each of the following **nursing interventions**, write an **expected patient outcome:**

1. Foley catheter removed at 1300 ⟹
2. Incentive spirometer q1h ×10 ⟹

CLINICAL SITUATION #2

Intershift report at 7:00 AM:

"The patient is 43 years old and was admitted 2 nights ago after experiencing GI bleeding. He is NPO and has an NG tube connected to continuous suction. The NG has drained 100 mL of dark reddish drainage. Vital signs at 6:00 AM are T 97.4° F, P 96, R 18, BP 130/86. A unit of whole blood is infusing and should be complete by 9:00 AM. His current Hgb is 8.6. He does have a history of ETOH abuse and has been more restless this morning."

The patient's current **flow charts** contain the following information:

Patient Care Kardex

IV: D_5/0.9 NS c̄ 10 mL MVI @ 100 mL/hr

IV site: #18 g LFA; saline lock RFA#20 g

Give two units of whole blood today ☑
H & H in the AM ☐

Routine Medication:
Mylanta 30 mL q4h/NG (clamp tube for 30 min after administration)
Famotidine 20 mg q12h IVPB 10-10

Intake and Output Record

Night Shift @ 0600

Intake			**Output**		
PO	=	0	UA void	=	525
			NG	=	100
IV	=	600			
0.9 NS	=	50			
Transfusion	=	50			

Interactive activity: With a partner, **use the case study and the flow charts** to:

1. Identify the pertinent patient information made known to you in the *report.*	2. Identify the pertinent patient information made known to you in the *flow charts.*	3. Review the data in columns 1 and 2 and identify information that needs follow-up.

THREE

It is 7:30 AM as you leave the report room. **Prioritize** your plan of care for the morning:

Time	Plan of Nursing Care

10:00 AM nursing assessment: Anxious, restless, pulled out NG tube. Physician called. Wrist restraints applied. VS: P 100, R 26, BP 146/90. Vomited 20 mL bright red fluid. Bowel sounds present ×4, abd. soft. Transfusion #2 infusing at 25 gtt/min.

The physician calls back and gives the following telephone orders:

Wrist and vest Posey restraints prn
Oxygen at 2 L/min/NP
Reinsert NG tube
ABG, serum electrolytes Mg^{++}, BG, Hgb & Hct
VS and neuro checks q2h
Librium 50 mg IM q3h prn restlessness
Phenergan 25 mg IM q4h prn N/V

1. Identify the nursing interventions that require immediate follow-up.	2. Identify the nursing actions that you can delegate/assign to unlicensed personnel.

For each of the following **nursing interventions**, write **expected patient outcomes:**

1. Application of wrist and Posey vest restraints ⟶
2. Librium 50 mg IM ⟶

CLINICAL SITUATION #3

Intershift report at 1600:

"The patient was admitted today for dehydration. She is 88 years old and has a stage IV pressure ulcer on her sacrum. A wet-to-dry dressing was applied. A pressure ulcer with eschar is on her left heel. She weighs 90 pounds and she refused her lunch. An IV was started at 1400. You have 750 mL credit. She is a sweet little lady, quiet, and at times forgetful. Her admission lab results just came in, her Hgb is 9.6, Hct 27, WBC 11,000, and K^+ 4.5. I have not called the physician."

The patient's current **flow charts** contain the following information:

Patient Care Kardex

VS q4h — Diet: Pureed
HOH
Siderails ↑ at all times
W-D Drsg $\bar{c}$ 0.9 NS 0600-1400-2200

IV: D_5/0.9 NS at 75 mL/hr
IV site: R hand #24 g cannula

Medication: Colace 100 mg daily

No Code

Intake and Output Record

Day Shift — 8 hour

Intake	Output
PO = 50	UA = inc ×2
IV = 250	

Interactive activity: With a partner, **use the case study and the flow charts** to:

1. **Identify the pertinent patient information made known to you in the *report.***	2. **Identify the pertinent patient information made known to you in the *flow charts.***	3. **Review the data in columns 1 and 2 and identify information that needs follow-up.**

It is 1630 as you leave the report room. **Prioritize** your plan of care for the next 4 hours:

Time	Plan of Nursing Care

At 2000 the nursing assistant reports that the patient is restless and trying to get out of bed. You document the following assessment: Speech incoherent, skin warm, flushed. VS: T 101° F, P 92, R 24, BP 108/60. Incontinent of dark-colored urine with strong odor. Physician called. The following telephone orders are given:

Catheterize for postresidual urine
VS q2h, I & O
Tylenol 325 mg po q4h prn T >100.4° F
Enc. fluid intake
Rocephin 1 g IVPB daily

1. Identify the nursing interventions that require immediate follow-up.	2. Identify the nursing actions that you can delegate/assign to unlicensed personnel.

For the following **nursing intervention**, write an **expected patient outcome:**

1. Monitor I & O q8h →

CLINICAL SITUATION #4

Intershift report at 2300:

"The patient was admitted with a fractured right tibia and is 1 day postop. He has a cast on. He has been quiet most of the evening. He just started coughing and is experiencing some SOB. He says he has a history of asthma and that he gets this way every now and then. I did not detect any wheezing. Vital signs are T 98.8° F, P 90, R 28, BP 140/88. Circulation, movement, and sensation are WNL in the right leg."

The patient's current **flow charts** contain the following information:

Nursing Care Rand

Diet: Regular

Up in chair
PT to teach crutch walking ☑

IV: Saline lock #20g RFA

Circ. movement, sensation and temp. (CMST) right leg q4h
Elevate leg on one pillow

PRN Medication:
PCA - morphine sulfate 1 mg/hr continuous; 1 mg/6 min/pt. demand; 4-hour limit = 30 mg

Medical History

Smokes ½ -1 pack of cigarettes/day

Respiratory infection 1 month ago
Uses cromolyn inhaler prn

CBC WNL } Day of admission
ESR ↑

48-yr-old male

Interactive activity: With a partner, **use the case study and the flow charts** to:

1. Identify the pertinent patient information made known to you in the *report*.	**2. Identify the pertinent patient information made known to you in the *flow charts*.**	**3. Review the data in columns 1 and 2 and identify information that needs follow-up.**

THREE

It is 2330 as you leave the report room. **Prioritize** your plan of care for the next 3 hours:

Time	Plan of Nursing Care

0200 nursing assessment: The patient is beginning to cough more frequently and complains of chest tightness. Respiratory assessment indicates inspiratory and expiratory wheezes in bilateral lungs. You call the physician and obtain the following telephone orders:

IV D5/0.9 NS at 125 mL/hr
Oxygen at 2 L/NP
Ventolin inhaler 2 puffs q4h
Alupent nebulizer treatment q3h
ABG, sputum for eosinophils
Solu-Medrol 125 mg IVP q6h
Check oxygen saturation with pulse oximeter q2h
Call physician with ABG results

1. Identify the nursing interventions that require immediate follow-up.	2. Identify the nursing actions that you can delegate/assign to unlicensed personnel.

For each of the following **nursing interventions**, write an **expected patient outcome:**

1. Alupent treatment q3h →
2. Solu-Medrol 125 mg IVP →

CLINICAL SITUATION #5

Intershift report at 3:00 PM:

"Mrs. C, 42 years old, was admitted earlier today with acute pancreatitis. She had mid epigastric pain with nausea and vomiting on admission. Her latest vitals signs are T 38° C, P 108, R 26, BP 110/60. Bowel sounds are hypoactive. I medicated her at 2:00 PM. A central line was inserted; you have 800 mL left in the IV. The NG is draining brownish fluid. She needs to have the urinary catheter inserted."

Mrs. C's current **flow charts** contain the following information:

Patient Care Kardex

VS: q4h Diet: NPO
O_2 @ 3 L/NP
Pulse oximetry q4h

IV: D_5W @125 mL/hr
Right central line
NG tube to low continuous suction ☑
Urinary catheter inserted ☐

ABG in AM ☐
K^+, Na^+, Cl^-, CO_2, Mg^{++}, Ca^{++} in AM ☐
Abd CT scan @ 6 PM today

Routine Medication:
Famotidine 20 mg q12h IVPB 10-10

PRN Medication:
Morphine sulfate 5 mg IV q3h prn pain

Admission Lab Data

Se Amylase	350 units/L
Se Lipase	260 units/L
Hgb	11.6 g/dl
Hct	32%
WBC	18,000/mm^3
LDH	300 units/L
AST	80 units/L
BG	200 mg/dl

Interactive activity: With a partner, **use the case study and the flow charts** to:

1. Identify the pertinent patient information made known to you in the *report.*	2. Identify the pertinent patient information made known to you in the *flow charts.*	3. Review the data in columns 1 and 2 and identify information that needs follow-up.

THREE

It is 4:00 PM; prioritize your plan of care for the next 3 hours:

Time	Plan of Nursing Care

At 8:30 PM the nursing assistant informs you that Mrs. C is complaining of pain and is restless. You note that she has not had a pain shot in the last 3 hours. You walk into the room to assess her and to give her the pain injection. She turns over quickly and pulls out the central line.

1. Identify the nursing interventions that you would implement immediately at the bedside.	2. Identify the follow-up nursing actions. Document the incident in the nurse's notes.

Nurse's Notes

For the following **nursing intervention**, write the **expected patient outcome:**

1. Call physician regarding abnormal lab values →

CLINICAL SITUATION #6

Intershift report at 8:00 AM:

"The patient is a young man who was transferred from the ICU yesterday. He was in a MVA 14 days ago. He had some head trauma and subsequent evacuation of a subdural hematoma. He is unconscious, unresponsive to painful stimuli, and flaccid. Pupils sluggish. He has several abrasions on his face and several bruised areas on his shoulders and chest from the accident. Vital signs are T 97.8° F, P 94, R 24, BP 124/80. Mother at bedside; she questions everything you do."

The patient's current **flow charts** contain the following information:

Nursing Care Rand

Suction prn — Diet: NPO
VS & Neuro checks q4h
Seizure precautions — Foley ☑
HOB ↑ 30° at all times — I & O
LBM: ______ — PEG tube clamped
IV: D_5/0.9% NS @ 100 mL/hr via right central line
Fingerstick BG q6h 12-6-12-6

Routine Medication:
Decadron 4 mg IVP q6h 10-4-10-4
Dulcolax supp. prn

Medical History

18-year-old high school student involved in a MVA in which he was the driver. Passenger in the car died from injuries. Pt. unconscious on arrival to the ER.

Drug use: Family not aware of any use. Blood alcohol level on admission 0.16%.

Family wants to continue all possible treatment. Not willing to discuss code status at this time.

Interactive activity: With a partner, **use the case study and the flow charts** to:

1. Identify the pertinent patient information made known to you in the *report.*	2. Identify the pertinent patient information made known to you in the *flow charts.*	3. Review the data in columns 1 and 2 and identify information that needs follow-up.

THREE

It is 8:30 AM as you leave the report room. **Prioritize** your plan of care for the next 3 hours:

Time	Plan of Nursing Care

2:00 PM nursing assessment: Pupil R • L • R. 12 Cheyne-Stokes. P 80, BP 150/80. Skin warm, jerky movements of the upper extremity noted. The physician writes the following orders:

Oxygen at 2 L/min/NP
Check oxygen saturation q1h
Vital signs q1h
CT scan stat
ABGs stat

1. Identify the nursing interventions that require immediate follow-up.	2. Identify the nursing actions that you can delegate/assign to unlicensed personnel.

For each of the following **nursing interventions**, write an **expected patient outcome:**

1. Oxygen 2 L/NP ⟶ ______
2. Seizure precautions ⟶ ______

CLINICAL SITUATION #7

Intershift report at 8:00 AM:

"The patient is 52 years old and has bone cancer. She has been requesting pain medication every 2 hours. I gave her morphine sulfate 2 mg this morning at 6:30 AM. Her respirations have gone down to 10 during the night. She does not want to be turned. A urinary catheter was inserted in the evening shift. She is a no code. A family member spent the night with her. Latest vital signs at 6:00 AM are T 97° F, P 66, R 12, BP 128/60."

The patient's current **flow charts** contain the following information:

Patient Care Kardex

Diet: DAT

VS q4h

Foley ☑

Comfort measures

I & O

IV: Saline lock

LBM: inc. ×1 sml

PRN Medication:

Morphine sulfate 2 mg IV q2h prn

Morphine sulfate 4 mg IV q2h prn if not relieved with morphine sulfate 2 mg

No code

Nurse's Notes

Night shift

11:00 PM Awake, responds when spoken to. c/o generalized pain, refuses to be turned. Morphine sulfate 2 mg IV given. – *C. Todd RN*

11:30 Resp 10, moans when touched, taking sips of water. Mouth care given. – *C. Todd RN*

12:00 AM Moaning. Daughter upset, crying, states is afraid that mother is going to die. Referral to pastoral care given. – *C. Todd RN*

1:00 2 mg morphine given, lethargic, arousable, resp. 10, P 60 BP 110/58. – *C. Todd RN*

4:30 Pain med. given —— *C. Todd RN*

5:00 Resting —— *C. Todd RN*

6:00 Lethargic but arousable —— *C. Todd RN*

Interactive activity: With a partner, **use the case study and the flow charts** to:

1. Identify the pertinent patient information made known to you in the *report.*	2. Identify the pertinent patient information made known to you in the *flow charts.*	3. Review the data in columns 1 and 2 and identify information that needs follow-up.

THREE

It is 8:30 AM as you leave the report room. **Prioritize** your plan of care for the next 3 hours:

Time	Plan of Nursing Care

At 12:30 PM you return from lunch to learn that the nursing assistant was unable to obtain a pulse on the patient. You assess the following: Unresponsive, skin cool, legs pale with mottling. Pulse not palpable, no apical pulse or BP audible. Family with patient. Physician contacted and pronounced patient.

Family is making arrangements for a mortuary to pick up the patient within the hour.

1. Identify the nursing interventions that require immediate follow-up.	2. Identify the nursing actions that you can delegate/assign to unlicensed personnel.

For each of the following **nursing interventions**, write an **expected patient outcome:**

1. Provide postmortem care → ______
2. Speak with family → ______

CLINICAL SITUATION #8

Intershift report at 7:00 AM:

"Mrs. F, 79 years old, was in a motor vehicle accident 2 days ago in which she fractured her arm. Her right arm is in a cast; circulation, movement, and sensation are fine. She is scheduled to go home this morning. She slept fine and was medicated for pain once during the night with relief."

At 7:30 AM, as you are coming out of report, the night nurse tells you that Mrs. F got up to go to the bathroom and fell going back to bed. She has a slight nosebleed and was given an icepack and assisted back to bed. The physician was called and informed of her falling. He said he would be in later to see her before discharge.

Mrs. F's current **flow charts** contain the following information:

Nursing Care Rand

VS: q shift Diet: DAT

LBM: 1 day ago

Discharge this AM.
Discharge instructions: Office appt. 2 wk
Vicodin tab i po q4h prn pain

PRN Medication:
Vicodin tab i po q4h prn pain
Benadryl 25 mg p.o. at bedtime prn q6h

Nurse's Notes

Night shift

11:00 PM Awake, oriented x3. Skin warm and dry. Pulse 88, slightly irregular, lung sound diminished bilaterally in the lower bases. Enc. to take deep breaths, used inspirometer x5. Right arm with cast, CMS-WNL. Requesting sleeping medication. Benadryl 25 mg po given. Side rails up. *S. Dolle RN*

1:30 AM Sleeping *S. Dolle RN*

4:30 AM Awake, requesting pain medication CMS-WNL. Vicodin tab i given *S. Dolle RN*

6:00 Resting comfortably. *S. Dolle RN*

Interactive activity: With a partner, **use the case study and the flow charts** to:

1. Identify the pertinent patient information made known to you in the *report.*	2. Identify the pertinent patient information made known to you in the *flow charts.*	3. Review the data in columns 1 and 2 and identify information that needs follow-up.

THREE

It is 7:30 AM; prioritize your plan of care for the next hour:

Time	Plan of Nursing Care

At 8:30 AM you note that Mrs. F is lethargic and very slow to respond to verbal stimuli. Skin is cool with slight cyanosis noted on nailbeds. P 110 irregular, R shallow, BP 90/70, which is lower than her usual of 130/88.

1. Identify the nursing interventions that you would plan to implement immediately.	2. Identify the nursing actions that you can delegate/assign to unlicensed personnel.

For each of the following **nursing interventions**, write an **expected patient outcome:**

1. Oxygen at 2 L/min/NP →
2. Insert saline lock →

CLINICAL SITUATION #9

Intershift report at 0700:

You are assigned to the following two patients:
"Mrs. A is 52 years old and has diabetes and hypertension. She is in for a pressure ulcer on her right heel. She is on bed rest with the right leg elevated and she only has BRP. There is a wet-to-dry dressing change due at 10. Her latest BP is 170/108."

"Mrs. C is 73 years old and was admitted with dehydration 3 days ago. She is eating and voiding normally. There is a possibility that she is going home today. I removed her saline lock; there was some redness at the site. She is not on any IV meds, so I decided not to restart. She says that she is going home late this afternoon, although there is no order. Her morning vital signs are T 97° F, P 82, R 8, BP 130/90."

Mrs. A's and Mrs. C's **medication records** contain the following information:

Medication Record

Routine	**Time**
Glyburide 10 mg po daily	0800
Tenormin 25 mg po daily	1100
(patient requests these hours)	
Furosemide 20 mg po bid	1100-1700
Cephalothin sodium IVPB q6h	10-4-10-4
PRN Medication	
MOM 30 mL prn constipation	
Restoril 30 mg po HS, may repeat x1	
Mrs. A	Allergies: None

Medication Record

Routine	**Time**
Minipress 1 mg po qAM	0900
Multivitamin tab i po qAM	0900
PRN Medication	
MOM 30 mL prn constipation	
Mrs. C	Allergies: None

Interactive activity: With a partner, **use the case study and the flow charts** to:

1. **Identify the pertinent patient information made known to you in the *report.***	2. **Identify the pertinent patient information made known to you in the *flow charts.***	3. **Review the data in columns 1 and 2 and identify information that needs follow-up.**
Mrs. A:	Mrs. A:	Mrs. A:
Mrs. C:	Mrs. C:	Mrs. C:

THREE

It is 0800; prioritize your plan of care for both patients for the next 3 hours:

Time	Plan of Nursing Care

You return from lunch at 1200 and Mrs. A is asking for her antihypertensive medication. You know you gave the medication, but she insists that you did not give her the medication. As you investigate, the nursing assistant tells you that Mrs. C is very lethargic and unresponsive. You suddenly realize that you gave Mrs. A's 1100 medications to Mrs. C.

1. Identify the nursing interventions that you would plan to implement immediately.	2. Make a nurse's note entry as to how you might document this incident.

For each of the following **nursing interventions**, write an **expected patient outcome:**

1. Prepare for a code →
2. Insert saline lock →

For a continuation of this case study, go to *http://evolve.elsevier.com/castillo/thinking.*

CLINICAL SITUATION #10

Intershift report at 11:00 PM:

"Mrs. J, 88 years old, was admitted this evening from a nursing home after the family found her lethargic and confused. Her admitting vital signs were T 101° F, P 92 and irregular, R 28 and short and shallow, BP 110/70. Her physician was called for admitting orders; he will come in tomorrow morning to see her. She was given Tylenol at 8:30 PM, and her current temperature is 100.6° F; she is still slightly confused. The family states that she had cataract surgery 1 week ago as an outpatient. She has an IV going. The patient in the next bed is concerned about Mrs. J's moaning."

Mrs. J's current **flow charts** contain the following information:

Nursing Care Kardex

VS q4h Diet: DAT

LBM: On admission
IV: 0.9% NS at 75 mL/hr
#24 angio cath RFA

Lab: CBC, Chem panel, UA

PRN Medication:
Tylenol 325 mg tabs ii q4h prn temp >101° F

Nurse's Notes from Skilled Nursing Facility

Documentation of latest nurse's notes:

1600 Turned, incontinent of urine, strong urine odor, incontinent pad applied. — *A. Cann LVN*
1700 Family in to visit. Upset, called physician. — *A. Cann LVN*
1830 Transferred to hospital per order. Recent UA culture reports show + MRSA. Unable to contact physician, copy of report included with transfer. — *T. Gage RN*

Interactive activity: With a partner, **use the case study and the flow charts** to:

1. Identify the pertinent patient information made known to you in the *report.*	2. Identify the pertinent patient information made known to you in the *flow charts.*	3. Review the data in columns 1 and 2 and identify information that needs follow-up.

It is 11:30 PM; prioritize your plan of care for the next hour:

Time	Plan of Nursing Care

Mrs. J is moved to a private room with isolation setup. She slept 1 to 2 hours at a time during the night and remains confused. She has developed a productive cough and is expectorating a small amount of thick, creamy, yellow-colored phlegm. Her morning vital signs are T 100.8° F, P 110, R 32, BP 114/82. At 6:30 AM the physician visits and leaves the following orders:

Vancomycin 500 mg q6h IVPB
Insert indwelling urinary catheter
Bed rest
Chest x-ray/ECG
Oxygen 2 L/min/NP, pulse oximeter q4h
I & O, enc. fluid intake

1. Identify the nursing interventions that you would plan to implement immediately.	**2. Identify the instructions you would give to staff and family in caring for Mrs. J.**

For the following **nursing intervention**, write an **expected patient outcome:**

1. Encourage fluid intake ⟹

CLINICAL SITUATION #11

Intershift report at 11:00 PM:

"The patient is 27 years old and was admitted this evening. He has been diagnosed with viral hepatitis. He is very jaundiced and his urine is very dark yellow. Intake for the shift was 100 mL and output 300 mL. He does not want to eat. He says he has not had an appetite for several days. The IV was started at 5:00 PM and is on time. His 8:00 PM vital signs are T 37.5° C, P 88, R 24, BP 130/70. He is currently complaining of itching and nausea. The lab reports just arrived and I put them in the patient's chart for the physician to see in the morning."

The patient's current **flow charts** contain the following information:

Nursing Care Kardex

VS: q4h — Diet: DAT
Bedrest c̄ BRP

Weigh daily ☑ — I & O

IV: D_5/0.9 NS @125 mL/hr
RFA # 22 g

Stool for occult blood ☐

PRN Medication:
Benadryl 50 mg capsule i q6h prn itching
Compazine 10 mg IM q6h prn N/V

Current Lab Data

AST 460 units/L
ALT 800 units/L
Alk Phosphatase 200 units/L

Hgb 12.0 g/dl
Hct 36%
WBC 10,000/mm^3

BS 160 mg/dl

PT 24 sec (Pt. control 12-16 secs)

Total bilirubin 14 mg/dl

Interactive activity: With a partner, **use the case study and the flow charts** to:

1. Identify the pertinent patient information made known to you in the *report.*	2. Identify the pertinent patient information made known to you in the *flow charts.*	3. Review the data in columns 1 and 2 and identify information that needs follow-up.

THREE

It is 11:30 PM; prioritize your plan of care for the next hour:

Time	Plan of Nursing Care

The patient is diagnosed with hepatitis A and is tentatively scheduled for discharge in 2 days.

1. Identify the dicharge information that you would include in teaching the patient and his family how best to recover from hepatitis A.

Diet: Fluids: Nausea/vomiting: Preventing transmission:	Activity: Skin care: Sexual concerns: Alcohol intake: Follow-up care:

For the following **nursing intervention**, write the **expected patient outcome:**

1. Patient education →

CLINICAL SITUATION #12

Intershift report at 7:00 AM:

"Mr. T, 67 years old, has prostate cancer with metastasis to the bone. I have medicated him around the clock for pain, the last dose given at 5:00 AM. He is lethargic but responds when spoken to. He needs frequent mouth care. His urine is amber. The 6:00 AM vital signs are stable at T 99° F, P 76, R 18, BP 126/74. Intake is 100 mL, output is 150 mL. His wife spent the night in the room and is making arrangements for hospice care."

Mr. T's current **flow charts** contain the following information:

Nursing Care Kardex

VS: q4h	Diet: Soft
Bed rest	
Saline lock ☑	I & O
RFA # 22 g	
Urinary catheter ☑	

PRN Medication:
Meperidine 100 mg q3h IVP prn pain

Allergies: Morphine sulfate

Pt: Mr. T — No code

Physician Progress Notes

Hosp. day #3

Assess: Skin warm, dry. T 99° F
↓ Oral intake
Output amber urine <600 mL/24 hr
Resp. diminished bilaterally

Alkaline phosphatase ↑
Acid phosphatase ↑

Plan: Keep comfortable
Hospice care being arranged
No code

Interactive activity: With a partner, **use the case study and the flow charts** to:

1. Identify the pertinent patient information made known to you in the *report.*	2. Identify the pertinent patient information made known to you in the *flow charts.*	3. Review the data in columns 1 and 2 and identify information that needs follow-up.

THREE

It is 7:30 AM; prioritize your plan of care for the next hour:

Time	Plan of Nursing Care

2:00 PM: Mrs. T calls to inform you that Mr. T is in a lot of pain and she is very upset and tells you that the pain shots do not seem to be giving him any comfort. You call the physician and suggest an order for something stronger. The physician orders morphine sulfate 15 mg IVP q3h prn pain. You administer the first dose at 2:15 PM. At 2:25 PM Mrs. T calls you into the room and tells you that her husband is not breathing.

On assessment, you note that Mr. T has stopped breathing and there is no pulse.

1. Identify the nursing interventions that require immediate follow-up.	2. Identify and discuss the ethical issue presented in this situation.

For the following **nursing intervention**, write the **expected patient outcome:**

1. Notify physician of patient's ⟹

CLINICAL SITUATION #13

Intershift report at 7:00 AM:

"Mrs. S, 58 years old, is 1 day postop right radical mastectomy. Her dressing is clean and dry. She has a Hemovac that drained 50 mL. Her vital signs at 6:00 AM are T 99.6° F, P 88, R 24, BP 150/90. She is using the PCA and a new IV liter was hung at 6:00 AM. Her right arm is elevated on a pillow; there is some swelling and she is complaining of some numbness."

Mrs. S's current **flow charts** contain the following information:

Nursing Care Kardex

VS: q4h	Diet: Clear liquid
Up in chair	I & O
IV: Lactated Ringer's @ 125 mL/hr	
LFA # 18 g	Hemovac ☑
Hgb & Hct this AM ☑	

Routine Medications:
Atenolol 50 mg po bid

PRN Medications:
PCA with morphine sulfate at 1 mg/6 min/pt. demand; not to exceed 30 mg in 4 hours

History and Physical

The patient is a 58-year-old female, widow. She lives alone. Does not smoke, drinks socially. Has mild hypertension 154/96.
Meds: Atenolol 50 mg po bid
Both parents deceased: mother died of breast cancer, father died of heart disease

Patient has two married daughters and one son

She found a hard lump in the right breast 3 weeks ago. A biopsy was done → Stage II
CEA 5 ng/mL

Plan: Right radical mastectomy
Chemotherapy to follow

Interactive activity: With a partner, **use the case study and the flow charts** to:

1. Identify the pertinent patient information made known to you in the *report*.	2. Identify the pertinent patient information made known to you in the *flow charts*.	3. Review the data in columns 1 and 2 and identify information that needs follow-up.

It is 7:30 AM; prioritize your plan of care for the next hour:

Time	Plan of Nursing Care

8:00 AM: You assess the following on Mrs. S: Alert and oriented. VS: T 99° F, P 94, R 28, BP 160/100. Lung sounds with fine crackles in the lower bases. Surgical dressing is clean and dry. Hemovac is compressed with 10 mL of reddish drainage. Right arm is elevated on a pillow. Finger puffy, c/o of a "numbness sensation." States on a 0-10 pain scale, the pain is at 2. Abdominal sounds present ×4. Antiembolic hose on. Lactated Ringer's infusing, site without redness or swelling, 500 mL left.

1. Identify the nursing interventions that require immediate follow-up.	2. Identify and discuss the postop educational needs of the patient.

For the following **nursing intervention**, write the **expected patient outcome:**

1. Encourage to participate in self-care activities →

CLINICAL SITUATION #14

Intershift report at 7:00 AM:

"Mr. S has left-sided heart failure. He had a restless night with some dyspnea and a dry nonproductive cough most of the night. Crackles are heard in both lungs. He has 3+ pitting edema in both legs and sacrum. His 6:00 AM vital signs are T 97.6° F, P 110 and irregular, R 34, BP 150/100. His IV site looks slightly puffy, but there is a good blood return. He just started to complain of nausea. His serum K^+ this morning is 3.0 mEq. It might be low because he is retaining fluid. His physician always comes in early so I posted the results in front of the patient's chart."

Mr. S's current **flow charts** contain the following information:

Nursing Care Kardex

VS: q4h	Diet: 2 g Na^+
↑ HOB	I & O
Bed rest with BRP	
Weigh daily ☑	
LBM (2 days ago)	
IV: D_5/0.45 NS $\bar{c}$ 20 mEq KCl	q12h
L hand # 20 g	
LAB:	
Digoxin level ☑	
K^+, Na^+, BUN, Creatinine, AST	☑
DX: Heart failure	Age: 72

Medication Record

Routine	Time
Digoxin 0.25 mg po qAM	0900
Furosemide 40 mg IVP BID	0900-1700
K-Dur 10 mEq po BID	0900-1700
Capoten 6.25 mg po TID	0900-1700-2200
Colace 100 mg po qAM	0900
PRN	
NTG SL 0.4 mg prn chest pain	

Interactive activity: With a partner, **use the case study and the flow charts** to:

1. Identify the pertinent patient information made known to you in the *report.*	2. Identify the pertinent patient information made known to you in the *flow charts.*	3. Review the data in columns 1 and 2 and identify information that needs follow-up.

THREE

It is 7:30 AM; prioritize your plan of care for the next hour:

Time	Plan of Nursing Care

9:00 AM: The physician has not come in to see Mr. S. Mr. S is alert but experiencing increasing shortness of breath, cough, and nausea and complaining of blurred vision. His pulse oximetry result is 88%. P 116 and irregular, R 34 and short and shallow, BP 152/100. Skin cool, color with slight cyanosis. Aside from the K^+ of 3.0 mEq, Mr. S's Na^+ is 135+ mEq, and his digoxin level is 2.4 ng/mL. You call the physician and learn that he is in surgery and will call you back within 30 minutes.

1. Identify the nursing interventions that require immediate follow-up.	2. Write a nurse's note to describe the 9:00 AM situation and the follow-up interventions.

For the following **nursing intervention**, write the **expected patient outcome:**

1. Lasix 40 mg IVP →

CLINICAL SITUATION #15

Intershift report at 7:00 AM:

"Mrs. LV, 74 years old, is 4 days postop left hip fracture. She had a Constavac that was removed yesterday. Surgical dressing is clean and dry. Pedal pulse on the left foot is present and the circulation, movement, and sensation are within normal limits. Lung sounds with fine crackles at the lower bases in both lungs. You need to encourage her to deep breathe and use the incentive spirometer. Her 6:00 AM vital signs are T 99.8° F, P 80, R 18, BP 130/82. She does not want to move, it seems like she is scared. I have medicated her two times during the night."

Mrs. LV's current **flow charts** contain the following information:

Nursing Care Kardex

VS: q shift — Diet: Soft
HOH — I & O
Ambulate with PT

LBM (2 days ago)

IV: Saline lock LFA #22 g angio cath
Inserted day of surgery

Routine Medications:

Digoxin 0.125 mg	po qAM	9
Furosemide 10 mg	po qAM	9
$FeSO_4$ 300 mg	po tid c̄ meals	8-12-5

PRN:
Vicodin tab q4h prn pain

Medical History

Elderly female brought into the ED after falling at home. A fracture of the left hip was diagnosed. She was taken to surgery and an ORIF was performed.
Hgb 9.4 mg/dl, Hct 28% on admission.

She lives alone, has one son and her husband died 2 years ago from a cardiac condition.

Patient has a history of atrial fibrillation.

THREE

Interactive activity: With a partner, **use the case study and the flow charts** to:

1. Identify the pertinent patient information made known to you in the *report*.	2. Identify the pertinent patient information made known to you in the *flow charts*.	3. Review the data in columns 1 and 2 and identify information that needs follow-up.

It is 7:30 AM; prioritize your plan of care for the next hour:

Time	Plan of Nursing Care

You review the nurse's notes from the night shift and note the following:

12:00 PM Alert, moaning, states leg hurts. Circulation, movement, and sensation of left leg WNL. Dressing clean and dry. Repositioned. Vicodin tab i given for pain.
2:00 AM Awake, states pain in leg, does not want to be touched. Left pedal pulse palpable. Repositioned.
4:00 AM Sleeping
6:00 AM c/o leg pain. Medicated with Vicodin tab i.

You enter the following assessment in the nurse's notes:

7:30 AM Awake, alert, states "did not have a good night." c/o leg pain. Left leg with pedal pulse, warm, cap. refill >2 sec. Leg elevated on pillow. Dressing clean and dry. Right leg with weak pedal pulse, swelling and redness noted at calf and thigh. Tender to touch. Lung sounds with fine crackles, encouraged to take deep breaths. Bowel sounds present ×4, c/o constipation.

1. Identify the nursing interventions that require immediate follow-up.	2. Identify the instructions that you will give the nursing assistants at this time.

For the following **nursing intervention**, write the **expected patient outcome:**

1. Elevation of right leg →

CLINICAL SITUATION #16

Intershift report at 3:00 PM:

"Mrs. L was admitted with signs and symptoms of having developed a pulmonary embolism. She just had a baby 2 weeks ago. She has a heparin drip. The infusion pump is set at 20 mL/hr. You have 100 mL left. She slept well. Respirations are unlabored at 22. The right lower lung has diminished breath sounds. She will be started on Coumadin today. She is anxious to go home and be with her baby."

Mrs. L's current **flow charts** contain the following information:

Nursing Care Kardex

VS: q4h Diet: Regular

Bed rest with BRP I & O
O_2 @ 3 L/min/NC prn SOB

IV: 500 mL D_5W $\bar{c}$ 20,000 units heparin
LFA #22 g angio cath
Infuse at 1000 units/hr

LAB:
Daily PTT ☑ PT in AM

Routine Medications:
Coumadin 5 mg po today at 0900
Coumadin 2.5 mg po today at 1700

Coagulation Record

Date	PTT	Control	Heparin dose
1st day	50 sec	25 sec	900 units/hr
2nd day	60 sec	25 sec	1000 units/hr
3rd day	90 sec	30 sec	1100 units/hr
Current	75 sec	30 sec	1000 units/hr

Interactive activity: With a partner, **use the case study and the flow charts** to:

1. Identify the pertinent patient information made known to you in the *report.*	2. Identify the pertinent patient information made known to you in the *flow charts.*	3. Review the data in columns 1 and 2 and identify information that needs follow-up.

THREE

It is 3:30 PM; **prioritize** your plan of care for the next hour:

Time	Plan of Nursing Care

6:30 PM The nursing assistant informs you that the IV pump is beeping. You go in to assess the pump and you notice that the heparin bag is empty. You look at the infusion pump and it is set at 35 mL/hr.

1. Identify the nursing interventions that require immediate follow-up.	2. Document your findings as you would enter them in the nursing notes.

For the following **nursing intervention**, write the **expected patient outcome:**

1. Monitor for signs and symptoms of bleeding →

CLINICAL SITUATION #17

Intershift report at 3:00 PM:

"Ms. P, 23 years old, had an emergency appendectomy yesterday. She has Down syndrome. She has gotten up to the chair twice today. Surgical dressing is clean, dry, and intact. Bowel sounds are hypoactive. Her IV is infusing well; you have 200 mL left. Oral intake is 100 mL and output is the 400 mL. I have medicated her at noon for pain. Her noon vital signs are T 100° F, P 80, R 20, BP 110/78."

Ms. P's current **flow charts** contain the following information:

Nursing Care Kardex

VS: q4h Diet: Clear liquid

Ambulate c̄ assistance I & O

IV: IL D_5/0.9 NS @ 125 mL/hr
LFA #22 g angio cath

Routine Medications:
Cefoxitin 2 g IVPB q6h 10 - 4 - 10 - 4

PRN Medications:
Morphine sulfate 8 mg IV q4h prn pain
Droperidol 1.25 mg IV q4h prn N/V

Intake and Output Record

7 – 3 shift:

Oral:	100	Void:	8:00 AM	50
			9:00	50
			11:00	75
			12:00	50
			1:00 PM	75
IV:	900		2:00	100
IVPB:	50			
		Emesis	12:00 PM	100
Total:	1050		Total:	500

Interactive activity: With a partner, **use the case study and the flow charts** to:

1. Identify the pertinent patient information made known to you in the *report.*	2. Identify the pertinent patient information made known to you in the *flow charts.*	3. Review the data in columns 1 and 2 and identify information that needs follow-up.

It is 3:30 PM; prioritize your plan of care for the next hour:

Time	Plan of Nursing Care

8:00 PM: Ms. P's mother and family are at the bedside. They tell you that Ms. P is increasingly restless and is pulling at her surgical dressing. You note the following entries in the nursing notes:

> Has voided a total of 100 mL since 4:00 PM. Emesis 100 mL greenish fluid at 6:00 PM, refused dinner. Morphine sulfate 8 mg and droperidol 1.25 mg given IV at 6:00 PM.

1. Identify the nursing interventions that require immediate follow-up.	2. Identify a rationale for each nursing intervention that you plan to implement.

For the following **nursing intervention**, write the **expected patient outcome:**

1. Ambulate patient →

CLINICAL SITUATION #18

Intershift report at 0700:

"Mr. O has cellulitis of the right leg. He is pretty much self-care and he says he is not used to being in bed so much. He stays in a chair most of the time with his leg elevated. His I & O is fine and his vital signs are stable at T 37° C, P 92, R 22, BP 164/94. He has a dry dressing on the right leg and there is no drainage. His saline lock needs to be changed today and his fingerstick blood glucose was 110 this morning."

Mr. O's current **flow charts** contain the following information:

Nursing Care Kardex

VS: q4h Diet: 2000 cal ADA
BRP
4x4 to right leg - Change q shift
LBM 1 day ago I & O
IV: Saline lock
LFA #22 g angio cath

Heating pad to right leg
Elevate leg on pillow

Fingerstick BG qAM 0600 ☑
C. O 62 yrs. Dx: Cellulits R. Leg
Hx: Angina, hypertension, DM type 2

Medication Record

Routine:

Glyburide 10 mg po qAM	0800	
Verapamil SR 240 mg po bid	0900	1700
Inderal 20 mg po bid	0900	1700
ASA 81 mg po qAM	0900	
Colace 100 mg po qAM	0900	

Velosef 2g IVPB q6h 2400-0600-1200-1800

PRN:
NTG SL 0.4 mg q5min ×3 prn chest pain

THREE

Interactive activity: With a partner, **use the case study and the flow charts** to:

1. Identify the pertinent patient information made known to you in the *report.*	**2. Identify the pertinent patient information made known to you in the *flow charts.***	**3. Review the data in columns 1 and 2 and identify information that needs follow-up.**

It is 0730; prioritize your plan of care for the next hour:

Time	Plan of Nursing Care

1200: Mr. O returns to bed after having a BM. You note that he is short of breath and his skin is cool and clammy. You assess his vital signs; his radial pulse is 110 and irregular, respirations are 32, and his BP is 170/100. He tells you that he is feeling pressure on his chest. You assist him into bed and place him in high-Fowler's position.

1. Identify your follow-up nursing interventions.	2. Identify a rationale for each nursing intervention that you plan to implement.

For the following **nursing intervention**, write the **expected patient outcome:**

1. Administration of oxygen →

CLINICAL SITUATION #19

Intershift report at 7:00 AM:

"Mr. I, 70 years old, is 1 day postop a TURP. He has a continuous normal saline irrigation. I will hang a new irrigation bag before I leave. He has had several clots during the shift. His vital signs are T 37.2° C, P 90, R 22, BP 160/93. He is alert and cheerful, and told me that he leads a very active life. I gave him a suppository for c/o bladder spasms at 5 this morning. The IV is also very positional."

Mr. I's current **flow charts** contain the following information:

Nursing Care Rand

VS q4h Diet: Clear liquids
Antiembolic hose on
LBM: On admission
IV: Lactated Ringer's at 75 mL/hr
#20 g angio cath RFA

3-way indwelling cath c̄ 30-mL balloon
NS continuous irrigation - keep UA free of clots

Routine Medication:
Colace 100 mg po qAM 1000
PRN Medication:
B & O supp. i q6h prn bladder spasms

Intake and Output Record

11-7 shift:

	Intake		Output
Oral:	50		1300
		(NS irrigation	1000)
IV:	300		
Total:	350		300

Interactive activity: With a partner, **use the case study and the flow charts** to:

1. Identify the pertinent patient information made known to you in the *report.*	2. Identify the pertinent patient information made known to you in the *flow charts.*	3. Review the data in columns 1 and 2 and identify information that needs follow-up.

THREE

It is 7:30 AM; prioritize your plan of care for the next hour:

Time	Plan of Nursing Care

8:00 AM: Mr. I is complaining of increased pain. He is grimacing, is diaphoretic, and tells you he has an urge to urinate. You note that the irrigation bag is empty and there are 50 mL of burgundy-colored urine in the urinary collection bag. There is urine leaking around the catheter.

1. Identify the nursing interventions that you would plan to implement immediately.	2. Identify the follow-up nursing interventions for the rest of the shift.

For the following **nursing interventions**, write an **expected patient outcomes:**

1. Bladder irrigation →
2. Encourage fluid intake →

CLINICAL SITUATION #20

Intershift report at 7:00 AM:

"Mrs. F, 46 years old, had a TAH-BSO yesterday. She had soft bowel sounds this morning. The abdominal dressing is clean and dry. Her IV is infusing well and she has an epidural infusion with fentanyl infusing through a pump. She has not had any breakthrough pain. The epidural dressing is intact and the catheter is fine. She has been mostly on bed rest, but she is to get up to a chair this morning. The 6:00 AM vital signs are T 37.5° C, P 78, R 18, BP 130/80. Her output was 500 mL."

Mrs. F's current **flow charts** contain the following information:

Nursing Care Rand

VS: q4h — Diet: Clear liquids
Up in chair with assistance
Incentive spirometer q1h ×10 WA
LBM: Prior to admission

Urinary catheter ☑

IV: D_5/0.45 NS q8h

Routine Medication:
Fentanyl in 6 mL/hr/pump NS via epidural catheter ordered by anesthesiologist

Intake and Output Record

Night shift:

Intake		Output	
Oral: (Sips of H_2O)	50	Void:	
		UA cath:	500
IV:	1000		
IV (Fentanyl):	48		

Interactive activity: With a partner, **use the case study and the flow charts** to:

1. Identify the pertinent patient information made known to you in the *report.*	2. Identify the pertinent patient information made known to you in the *flow charts.*	3. Review the data in columns 1 and 2 and identify information that needs follow-up.

THREE

It is 7:30 AM; prioritize your plan of care for the next hour:

Time	Plan of Nursing Care

At 8:30 AM: Mrs. F gets up with assistance to sit in a chair. As she walks slowly to the chair, she steps on some of the tubings. The nursing assistant tells you that the infusion pump is beeping. You go in to assess and note that the epidural infusion pump is beeping and the patient's epidural dressing is pulled from the patient's back. The epidural catheter seems to be pulled out.

1. Identify the nursing interventions that you would plan to implement immediately.	2. Document your findings as you would enter them in the nursing notes.

For the following **nursing intervention**, write an **expected patient outcome:**

1. Cover epidural site with 4 × 4 ⟹

CLINICAL SITUATION #21

The nurse reviews the history and physical (H & P) and the care plan of the assigned patient:

Admitting Information: Mr. W, 72-year-old male of Chinese descent. Brought into the office by his son. The son provided most of the information because the patient speaks little English. The patient lives in China but has been in the U.S. for 5 months visiting his son. He was planning to return home in a couple of weeks.

Physical Examination:

VS. T 99.8° C, P 92, R 28, BP 130/90, Pulse oximetry 94%

Neuro: Alert, soft-spoken, smiles and answers questions appropriately via the son, who interprets. PERRLA.

Resp: Rhonchi bilaterally. Productive cough with yellow-colored phelgm. Dyspnea. Indicates that "chest hurts all over."

CV: Pulse slightly irregular. Murmur—neg.

Integ: Dry, decreased turgor.

GI: Abdomen soft, nontender. Son states his father is not eating very well. He misses the traditional cooking but does like some American soups. Denies constipation.

GU: No complaints. WNL.

Psychosocial: Quiet, small frame, thin man.

Medications: Prescription medications—none. Has been using several herbal teas for "the cold in his chest."

Day Shift Report to Evening Shift: Mr. W has been in the hospital for 2 days. There is always someone in the room with the patient. His son spent the night with him.

The patient is quiet and speaks little English. He seems to respond better to male nurses. Lung sounds are still diminished in the lower bases. Has refused his bath for 2 days now. He has lost another pound since admission. His IV is infusing well at 125 mL/hr.

Day Shift Nursing Notes:

0800 Neuro: Awake, quiet, and cooperative. PERRL.
Resp: Diminished in the lower bilateral bases. Productive cough with light yellowish sputum. Pulse ox 94%. SOB noted. O_2 at 2 L/NC.
CV/Skin: Warm, cap refill <3 sec. Turgor non-elastic.
GI: Active bowel sounds x4 quadrants. — N. Nurse RN

0900 GI: Ate 50% of breakfast. Family has brought in some food for the patient.
MS: Up to bathroom with assistance from the son. SOB noted on exertion. Son states that the father is upset because he believes his urine smells bad because of the IV medication. — N. Nurse RN

1300 GI: Ate 10% of lunch. Drinking teas and soups brought from home. — N. Nurse RN

1400 Systems unchanged. — N. Nurse RN

Interactive activity: With a partner, **use the case study and the flow charts** to:

1. Identify the pertinent *cultural information* made known to you from the H & P.	2. Identify the cultural data you gathered from the *report and nursing notes.*	3. List the *cultural considerations* that influence health care delivery.

THREE

Use the **Cultural Considerations** listed in the left-hand box below to develop **realistic nursing interventions** that demonstrate culturally sensitive care for Mr. W:

Cultural Considerations	**CARE PLAN**
• Communication • Food preferences • View of health care practitioner role • Patient's role in the family • Patient's view of Western medicine with regard to current illness • Patient's view of what caused the illness • Patient's view of what would be beneficial for getting better	Interventions:

On the third hospital day, Mr. W refuses the 0800 dose of IV Cefizox and refuses to let the nurse listen to his lungs. He tells the family that he is tired and wants to be left alone. His 0800 VS are T 98.9° F, P 96, R 26, BP 134/90, pulse oximetry 84%.

1. Identify the nursing interventions that you would implement at this time.	**2. Identify a rationale for each intervention that you plan to implement.**

For the following **nursing diagnosis**, write an **expected outcome:**

1. Risk for Injury ⟹

CLINICAL SITUATION #22

Mr. S, 46 years old, comes into the urgent care center with complaints of fatigue, muscle aches, a cough, and sweating. Vital signs are T 99.8° F, P 90, R 28, BP 130/88. Mr. S tells the nurse that he has had these symptoms for the last 48 hours and that he cannot afford to be ill. He says that he has a lot of work waiting for him at the office because there have been rumors regarding anthrax exposure of several persons from one of the government buildings several blocks away. The information obtained from Mr. S includes:

Examination	Familial History	Social History
Neuro: A/O c/o slight headache. Resp: Rhonchi bilaterally. Nonproductive cough, SOB noted. C/o sore throat and chest area "a little sore." CV: Regular pulse, heart sounds WNL. GI: Anorexia. Abdomen soft, nontender. GU: WNL.	Married, 2 children, both healthy (1 male, 15 years; 1 female, 12 years). Wife works as a secretary part-time. Mother: Deceased; trauma from an auto accident. Father: DM type 2, hypertension. **Employment History** Government employee for 15 years.	Alcohol: Drinks occasionally Medications: Vitamins, echinacea tablets (heard it helped in decreasing the effects of a cold). Activities: Golfs twice a month, gym (weights and treadmills). Describes himself as a "generally healthy person."

Interactive activity: With a partner, **use the case study and the flow charts** to:

1. **Identify the pertinent patient information made known to you from the *signs and symptoms*.** →	2. **Identify the pertinent information you gathered from the *patient history*.** →	3. **Review the data in columns 1 and 2 and identify information that needs follow-up.**

The patient is diagnosed and admitted to the acute-care setting with signs and symptoms of inhalation anthrax. Read the **physician orders** below and **write a rationale** for each order:

Physician Orders	
1. Contact isolation	**1. Contact isolation:**
2. Chest x-ray stat	**2. Chest x-ray stat:**
3. VS q4h with neuro checks	**3. VS q4h with neuro checks:**
4. CBC, 12-Chem panel, UA	**4. CBC, 12-Chem panel, UA:**
5. Cipro 400 mg IVPB now	**5. Cipro 400 mg IVPB now:**

At 1600 the nursing assistant reports the following: T 99° F, P 120, R 30, BP 118/80, pulse oximetry 92%. The patient was difficult to arouse.

1. Identify the nursing interventions that you would plan to implement immediately.	2. Identify a rationale for each nursing intervention that you plan to implement.

For the following **nursing interventions**, write an **expected outcome:**

1. Notify immediate family. ⟶
2. Notify pastoral care. ⟶

Section Four - Management and Leadership

MANAGEMENT AND LEADERSHIP CLINICAL SITUATION #1

The supervisor of a medical unit has recently hired several new RNs just out of nursing school. Two of the new RNs have started on the day shift. As an RN with 7 years of experience, you have been assigned to orient and precept one of the new RNs. The new RN will work with you for 3 months.

Information about the experienced RN: You have worked mainly on the medical unit and are considered an expert. You are always on time. You are organized and can be counted on "to get the job done." You are frequently given all the new employees to orient. You have never complained and you like working with nurses, but you are getting pretty tired of having to be the one that is assigned to orient the new employees all the time.

Information about the new RN: He is in his twenties, quiet but friendly. He works steadily, has a good knowledge base, but has difficulty asking questions. He has managed the care of three patients in school. He was late the first day on the unit and tells the nurse that he "is more of a night person."

1. Identify the strong and weak characteristics demonstrated in the RNs.

Strong characteristics of the experienced RN	Weak characteristics of the experienced RN	Strong characteristics of the new RN	Weak characteristics of the new RN

2. Prioritize the one major issue that may cause conflict initially.

1. ______________________

As the experienced RN, how would you handle this major issue?

____

Before implementing the plan, what other issues should be considered?

____

FOUR

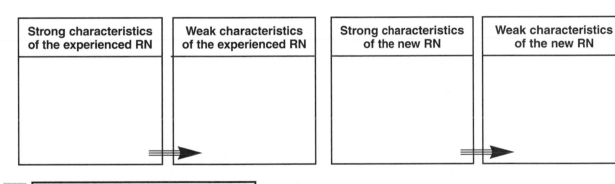

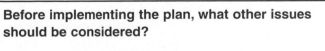

Clinical situation continued:

As the experienced nurse, you develop the following goals to help guide the progress of the new RN. You discuss these goals with the new RN.

Goals for the first week:	Goals for the second week:

At the end of the 2 weeks, the new RN has not been able to achieve the set goals. The experienced RN sets up a time to meet with the new RN. During the meeting, the new RN is visibly upset.

1. Identify the issues that may be affecting the new RN

Issues:

____

____

____

____

____

____

****

With a partner, role play the part of the experienced nurse and the new RN.

As the experienced RN, how would you handle this situation?	As the new RN, how would you like this situation handled?

MANAGEMENT AND LEADERSHIP CLINICAL SITUATION #2

The hospital administration has decided to implement a new computerized charting program to be used in all of the nursing units for charting patient assessments. For the last 6 months the staff has been required to attend computer training classes offered at the hospital. Training manuals and informational flyers have been placed in all the units. Talk and rumors about this new change has taken place for months, but no one actually believed that it would happen. Now the units seem chaotic as the technology staff install the new computers while the nurses work around them to provide patient care.

Information about administration's decision: The computerized program has been studied for months. Charge nurses and staff nurses from all shifts have been involved in evaluating the program and giving feedback. The administration has invested time and money into this form of charting and is committed to implementing this program throughout the hospital. Computerized training will be mandatory for all nurses.

Information about the staff: The implementation of the new charting format has brought about mixed feelings among the staff. The younger nurses are excited and think that the charting will be "fun." The older nurses feel that it will take more time and do not understand how the new computerized program will make charting easier. Comments from nurses range from "Isn't this exciting?" to "The administration can spend thousands of dollars in these computers but has a hard time giving us a raise when we are the ones doing all the work." The managers, supervisors, and charge nurses are asked to support this change and to ensure that all staff are trained.

1. Identify the issues/reactions from the different levels.

Hospital Administration	Managers, Supervisors, and Charge Nurses	Staff

How do the clinical situation and the staff's comments and feelings correlate with the change process?

FOUR

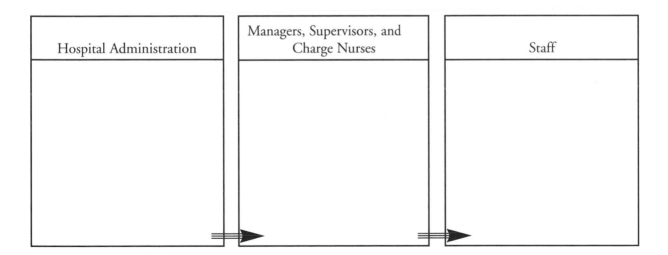

Clinical situation #2 continued:

You are the charge nurse of the unit that has been selected to be the first one to use the new computerized program. Some staff members are very excited to be the first ones to use the program and other staff members are requesting to transfer to another unit. Administration has asked you to ensure that the staff use the program and to identify how the administrative staff can help you facilitate the implementation of this computerized program on your unit.

1. Identify strategies that can help you implement the change and help your staff cope with the change. →	**2. Identify specific requests that can guide administration in helping you and your staff implement this change.**

How does the development of strategies, both for staff and administration, help with the process of change?

____

____

****

After 2 weeks of using the program, your most experienced nurse requests to be transferred to a unit that is not using the computer program. You, the charge nurse, know that all the units will be using the computer program within the next 6 months. The nurse is very good and you do not want to lose her.

With a partner, role play the part of the nurse and the charge nurse.

As the charge nurse, how would you handle this situation?	As the nurse, how would you like this situation handled?

MANAGEMENT AND LEADERSHIP CLINICAL SITUATION #3

An RN is transferred to the medical unit after working 5 years in the intensive care unit. It has taken some time—3 months to be exact—to organize and manage the care of 4 to 5 patients assigned to her on the day shift. The majority of the patients are high acuity with multiple problems. Most of the staff have been very supportive, always checking to see whether they can help. However, the RN has observed one nursing assistant who rarely helps out the other staff members. The RN also believes that some interventions by the nursing assistant have been performed incorrectly.

Information about the RN: The RN is used to working independently. She would rather do the procedure or provide the care herself to ensure that it is done correctly. This has been a difficult transition for her because she has to rely on ancillary help to complete her work. Although the RN can delegate many tasks, she finds herself avoiding this nursing assistant and mostly doing the tasks herself. She stays late everyday to complete the charting on the patients.

Information about the nursing assistant: The nursing assistant has been on this unit for 1 year. She feels pretty comfortable with her skills and has even shown other nursing assistants how to take short cuts. She enjoys working by herself and takes pride in not asking anyone for help. She does not like being told how to do something that she already knows how to do. She is frustrated with the RN because the RN seems to be running around in circles. As far as she is concerned, she will do her job, and, unless asked, she will not do anything extra.

1. Identify the characteristics demonstrated in the RN that interfere with effective delegation.

In managing this situation, what can the RN do to work with the problem and create a more conducive working environment with the nursing assistant?

___

___

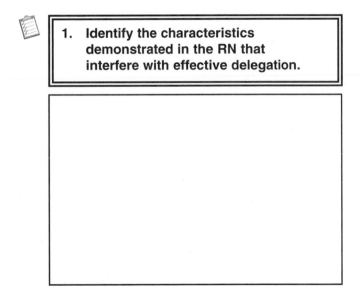

Clinical situation #3 continued:

The following day the nursing assistant is assigned to work with the RN. There are numerous tasks that need to be done on the patients. The nurse has the following tasks that need to be done for the assigned patients: vital signs, three bed baths, assessments, saline lock irrigations, emptying urinary collection bags on two patients, emptying a J-P device, W-D dressing change, passing narcotic medications, applying restraints, monitoring IV fluids, NG tube bolus feeding, oral suctioning, deep suctioning, pulse oximetry, starting oxygen per nasal cannula.

1. List the tasks that need to be performed by the RN.	**2. List the tasks that may be delegated to the nursing assistant.**

List the criteria that should be considered before delegating a task to another person.

____

____

****

After the RN has taken her own noon vital signs, the nursing assistant approaches her and asks her why she did not let her take the noon vitals on the patients.

With a partner, role-play the part of the RN and the nursing assistant.

As the RN, how would you problem-solve this situation?	As the nursing assistant, what would you like to come out of this situation?

MANAGEMENT AND LEADERSHIP CLINICAL SITUATION #4

Two RNs have worked the day shift together on the oncology unit for several years. Both are expert nurses and through the years they have become close personal friends. RN Nurse A has accepted the position of charge nurse of the oncology unit, and RN Nurse B continues as a staff nurse. For the last 6 months, the charge nurse has been concerned about numerous discrepancies in the narcotics count. Lately, an increasing number of patients have been complaining that they are not obtaining pain relief after being medicated. After a careful investigation by the administrative staff, it was noted that all the narcotic count discrepancies occurred on the day shift. RN Nurse A is the only person informed of the current findings. A follow-up investigation will be conducted.

Information about RN Nurse A: The RN is married and has two children. She is frequently involved with the school activities of the children. She loves the staff and enjoys her work but is still learning the duties of a manager. She has a difficult time supervising and evaluating staff and seems to avoid handling any conflict situations. She has noticed that RN Nurse B has been irritable but has assumed that her marital separation is contributing to her behavior. After assessing the behaviors of RN Nurse B, she is wondering whether her friend may be involved with the narcotic discrepancies.

Information about RN Nurse B: The RN has two children in school and has recently separated from her husband. She has been unable to be active in her children's school activities because of the added demands brought on by the separation. She has been suffering from migraine headaches but cannot afford to miss any work because the couple had just purchased a new home before the separation. She has asked RN Nurse A to assign her to extra shifts or overtime whenever possible.

1. Identify the responsibility of RN Nurse A to the employer at this time.	→	2. Identify the responsibility of RN Nurse A to RN Nurse B at this time.

RN Nurse A feels that she is not being honest with the staff by not sharing the preliminary findings of the investigation. Identify issues that should be considered in this situation.

____

____

FOUR

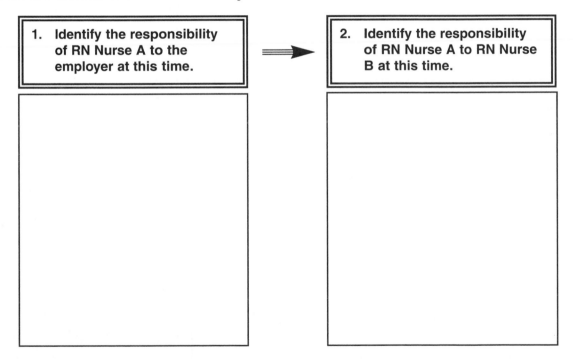

Clinical situation #4 continued:

For 3 weeks the narcotic count has been correct. Today, RN Nurse B is assigned to a terminally ill patient. She is preparing to administer pain medication to a patient and takes a syringe labeled morphine sulfate 10 mg from the narcotic drawer. She administers the medication IV to the patient. Thirty minutes later the patient is moaning with pain, and the family is very upset seeing him in such pain. The physician is called, and an order for a stat dose of morphine sulfate 5 mg IV is given. RN Nurse A administers the drug to the patient because RN Nurse B is at lunch. The patient is calm for the next 2 hours. RN Nurse A informs RN Nurse B about the additional dose of pain medication given to the patient. At the end of the shift, there is a discrepancy with the morphine sulfate and the narcotic count.

1. Identify the responsibility of RN Nurse A to the employer at this time.

2. Identify the responsibility of RN Nurse A to RN Nurse B at this time.

****

The next day, RN Nurse B is again preparing to administer morphine sulfate 10 mg IV to the patient. RN Nurse B emptied the contents of the morphine sulfate into another syringe and put this syringe in her pocket. She then filled the current syringe with saline solution and took this syringe into the room and gave the saline solution to the patient.

RN Nurse A noticed that RN Nurse B had a syringe with liquid in her pocket as she was going home. RN Nurse A confronts RN Nurse B. RN Nurse B tells her friend that it is saline solution, but she refuses to discard it or to give it to RN Nurse A.

With a partner, role-play the part of the RN Nurse A and the RN Nurse B.

As RN Nurse A, how would you handle this situation?

As RN Nurse B, what would you like to come out of this situation?

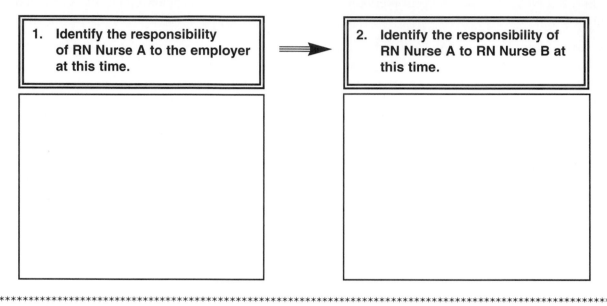

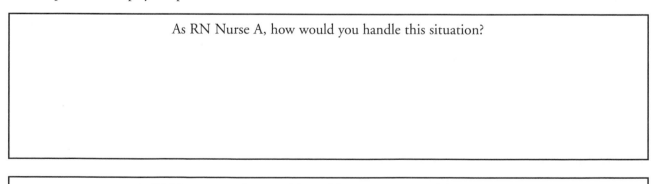

MANAGEMENT AND LEADERSHIP CLINICAL SITUATION #5

The RN works on an endocrine unit in a hospital that uses a team approach to deliver patient care. The team consists of an RN, an LVN, and two nursing assistants. The RN is responsible for the supervision and the delegation of care. A new, highly recommended LVN has recently been hired to work on the unit. During the first week of orientation, the supervising RN noticed that the LVN was friendly but did not check the insulin dosages with anyone before giving the insulin injections to the patients. The RN told the LVN to have all insulin dosages double-checked before giving. The LVN told one of the nursing assistants that the RN did not trust her. Later, the RN again saw the LVN giving an insulin injection to another patient without checking the insulin dose. The RN questioned the LVN, and the LVN coldly responded that she forgot because she never had to have her worked checked in her previous job and she would try to remember next time.

Information about the RN: The RN has been working on the endocrine unit for 2 years. She is very conscientious and, because she has diabetes mellitus, she takes a special interest in working with patients who have diabetes. She works closely with her staff and has not had any serious staff problems. She can tell that the LVN has a lot of experience and is willing to work with her. The RN has little patience for what she considers "unsafe practice" behaviors.

Information about the LVN: The LVN has been a nurse for 15 years. She has worked in several hospitals. In her last job, she worked in a skilled facility where she had increased responsibility. She decided to return to the acute care setting because it offered better financial benefits. She feels that she has a lot of experience and knows more than some of the new RNs. She can tell that the staff RN is recently out of school.

1. Identify the strong and weak characteristics demonstrated in each nurse.

Strong characteristics of the RN	Weak characteristics of the RN	Strong characteristics of the LVN	Weak characteristics of the LVN

2. Prioritize the major issue that needs to be addressed at this time.

1. ______________________

As the RN, how would you handle this situation?

____

FOUR

Clinical situation #5 continued:

For the next 2 weeks, the RN noticed that the LVN had been double-checking the insulin dosages. Today, the unit is very busy and one patient in particular is very upset and requested to speak with the RN. The patient complained of several things but was especially upset because the LVN was going to give him the wrong dose of insulin this morning. The patient explained that he asked the LVN how much insulin she was giving him and that she said 10 units of NPH. The patient insisted that he normally was given 12 units of NPH every morning. The LVN checked, and the patient was correct.

The RN discussed the patient's comments with the LVN. The LVN agreed with the patient's comments, telling the RN that it really wasn't a big issue because the dose was a little less than ordered and it could have easily been corrected. The RN decided to set up a meeting with the LVN to discuss the incident further and to present the following anecdotal note:

12/31 0900 Patient X complained that the LVN was going to administer 10 units of NPH insulin to him this morning instead of the usual 12 units he gets every morning. The LVN rechecked the ordered amount and proceeded to administer the correct dose to the patient.

I have told the LVN to double-check all insulin dosages before administering the injection to the patients. The LVN does not realize the seriousness of this behavior.

Discuss, evaluate, and rewrite the anecdotal note.

Anecdotal notes should contain:

****

The RN meets with the LVN.

With a partner, role-play the part of the RN and the LVN.

As the RN, how would you handle this situation?

____

____

____

____

____

____

____

____

Identify key points to keep in mind when conducting an evaluation meeting with an employee.

MANAGEMENT AND LEADERSHIP CLINICAL SITUATION #6

The medical unit staff of an acute-care hospital includes several RNs who have worked on this unit for more than 10 years. In addition to caring for higher-acuity patients, the nurses on the medical unit have also seen a change in the cultural makeup of the staff. The hospital has recently hired six new RNs from various ethnic backgrounds: two Middle Eastern nurses, one Chinese nurse, one Korean nurse, one Hispanic nurse, and one male nurse from Nigeria. All the nurses were trained outside the United States and were successful in passing the NCLEX-RN examination. Although all the nurses have taken additional classes and training, this is the first full-time job in the acute-care setting.

After going through the regular hospital orientation, the nurses are assigned to work on the day and evening shifts. After 2 months, three of the female nurses are having great difficulty working on the medical unit. Several of the regular RNs are complaining that the new nurses are not as competent and that they do not know how to relate with the staff and with the patients. Several staff members have asked to be transferred to another unit.

The unit manager solicited input from the new RNs and the regular staff and was told the following:

Comments made from the new RNs:

- Do not feel they are viewed as competent RNs.
- Staff members are impatient with them and take over tasks instead of letting them learn the tasks.
- Unlicensed personnel do not come to them with patient problems.
- General comments are made that make them feel incompetent.
- Have even been told to "speak English" several times.
- Their names have been changed to names that the staff can easily pronounce.
- There are a couple of RNs and staff members who are sympathetic and helpful.

Comments made from the regular RNs and staff:

- Change-of-shift reports are difficult to understand.
- Interactions with patients are minimal and not personal.
- The new RNs require a lot of guidance and still leave many tasks for the other shifts.
- The new RNs are afraid to approach physicians or to call physicians for orders.

FOUR

1. List the primary issues as viewed by the new RNs.

2. List the primary issues as viewed by the regular RNs and staff.

Clinical situation #6 continued:

Analyze the issues presented and list the management and cultural issues that need to be addressed.

Management-Related Issues/Needs	Culturally Related Issues/Needs

List management strategies that should be considered to address the issues presented:

In the clinical setting, it is important to become aware of cultural communication (tone of voice, use of words, gestures, touch, nonverbal communication) with staff and peers.

With a partner, identify cultural beliefs and values seen among peers and staff in the clinical setting. Discuss clinical examples and the implications related to health care delivery.

Possible cultural beliefs and values:

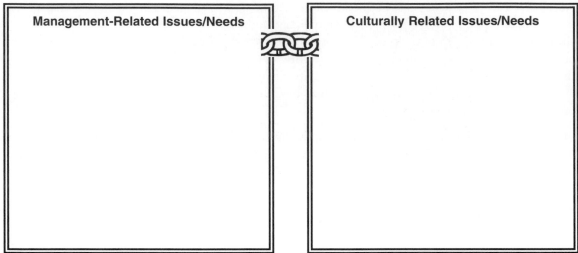

Section Five - Applying Critical Thinking Skills to Test Questions

APPLYING CRITICAL THINKING SKILLS TO TEST QUESTIONS

INSTRUCTIONS: **Circle the one best answer for each test question.** Write your rationale for selecting the answer. To enhance your learning and test-taking skills, discuss your answer and rationale with a partner. The answer and the rationale can be found on the back of this page.

1. The nurse is demonstrating how to minimize occlusion of a feeding tube after medication administration. Which nursing intervention is most important to include in the demonstration?
   a. Withdraw any residual, give the medication, and flush with 30 mL of water.
   b. Flush the tube with 20 mL of water before and after giving the medication.
   c. Use 30 mL of lukewarm water to flush the tube after giving the medication.
   d. Inject 15 mL of air before and after giving the medication.

Rationale: ______________________________

2. The client is discharged on phenytoin (Dilantin) 100 mg po due at 0800-1600-2400 and an antacid 30 mL prn. For effective drug administration, discharge instructions should include:
   a. Administer the phenytoin with a dose of antacid.
   b. Skip a dose of the phenytoin if the antacid is taken.
   c. Take half the dose of antacid if given with the phenytoin.
   d. Avoid taking the antacid at the same time as the phenytoin.

Rationale: ______________________________

3. The client is receiving total parenteral nutrition through a single-lumen central catheter per infusion pump. Ceftriaxone 1 g in 100 mL 0.9% NaCl is ordered daily IVPB. To safely administer this IVPB, the nurse plans to:
   a. administer the IVPB through a Y-port tubing above the infusion pump.
   b. administer the IVPB through a Y-port tubing below the infusion pump.
   c. start a peripheral line for the IVPB.
   d. use a mini-drip tubing for the IVPB.

Rationale: ______________________________

APPLYING CRITICAL THINKING SKILLS TO TEST QUESTIONS

HELPFUL HINTS: Read all test questions carefully. Identify key words in the question that will guide you in answering the question. In these test questions the **key words** to consider are **"most important," "effective drug administration,"** and **"safely."** Compare your rationale with the one in the test question.

1. The nurse is demonstrating how to minimize occlusion of a feeding tube after medication administration. Which nursing intervention is most important to include in the demonstration?
   a. Withdraw any residual, give the medication, and flush with 30 mL of water.
   (b.) Flush the tube with 20 mL of water before and after giving the medication.
   c. Use 30 mL of lukewarm water to flush the tube after giving the medication.
   d. Inject 15 mL of air before and after giving the medication.

Rationale: The answer is (b). It is important to initially check the placement of the nasogastric tube to ensure that the tube and suction are working. Options (a), (c), and (d) do not present the proper technique for administering medications through a feeding tube.

2. The client is discharged on phenytoin (Dilantin) 100 mg po due at 0800-1600-2400 and an antacid 30 mL prn. For effective drug administration, discharge instructions should include:
   a. Administer the phenytoin with a dose of antacid.
   b. Skip a dose of the phenytoin if the antacid is taken.
   c. Take half the dose of antacid if given with the phenytoin.
   (d.) Avoid taking the antacid at the same time as the phenytoin.

Rationale: The answer is (d). Absorption of phenytoin may be decreased when it is taken with an antacid. Options (a) and (c) do not address the effects of an antacid on phenytoin. Drug therapy should not be altered; therefore, option (b) is not correct.

3. The client is receiving total parenteral nutrition through a single-lumen central catheter per infusion pump. Ceftriaxone 1 g in 100 mL 0.9% NaCl is ordered daily IVPB. To safely administer this IVPB, the nurse plans to:
   a. administer the IVPB through a Y-port tubing above the infusion pump.
   b. administer the IVPB through a Y-port tubing below the infusion pump.
   (c.) start a peripheral line for the IVPB.
   d. use a mini-drip tubing for the IVPB.

Rationale: The answer is (c). IVPBs cannot be administered in a TPN line. Options (a) and (b) do not safely administer the IVPB because the TPN is used. Option (d) can be used but does not identify how the IVPB will be administered.

APPLYING CRITICAL THINKING SKILLS TO TEST QUESTIONS

INSTRUCTIONS: Circle the one best answer for each test question. Write your rationale for selecting the answer. To enhance your learning and test-taking skills, discuss your answer and rationale with a partner. The answer and the rationale can be found on the back of this page.

1. The nurse learns in report that the serum potassium level of a client is 5.5 mEq/L this morning. The client's physician is in surgery, so a message is left at the physician's office. The client is on the following medications at 0800: famotidine (Pepcid) 20 mg po and spironolactone (Aldactone) 50 mg po. Which action by the nurse is most appropriate?
   a. Hold the morning dose of famotidine until the physician returns the call.
   b. Hold the morning dose of spironolactone until the physician returns the call.
   c. Hold all the morning medications until the physician returns the call.
   d. Give all the morning medications as ordered.

Rationale: ____

____

____

____

____

2. The nurse is caring for a client with diabetes mellitus type 2. The following medications are listed on the client's medication record: metformin (Glucophage) 0.5 g po bid and repaglinide (Prandil) 1 mg po with meals. The morning blood glucose fingerstick is 98 mg/dl. Which action by the nurse is most appropriate?
   a. Hold the morning po medications.
   b. Give the metformin but hold the repaglinide.
   c. Give the repaglinide but hold the metformin.
   d. Give the po medications as ordered.

Rationale: ____

____

____

____

____

3. The client with end-stage renal disease is scheduled for hemodialysis in 2 hours. He has a (L) AV fistula and needs assistance with feeding. In delegating the care of the client, which nursing order is of priority?
   a. Feed the client first.
   b. Give all morning care before the dialysis.
   c. Take the blood pressure in the right arm.
   d. Feel for a vibration on the left arm.

Rationale: ____

____

____

____

____

FIVE

APPLYING CRITICAL THINKING SKILLS TO TEST QUESTIONS

HELPFUL HINTS: Read all test questions carefully. Identify key words in the question that will guide you in answering the question. In these test questions the **key words** to consider are "**most appropriate**" and "**priority.**" Compare your rationale with the one in the test question.

1. The nurse learns in report that the serum potassium level of a client is 5.5 mEq/L this morning. The client's physician is in surgery, so a message is left at the physician's office. The client is on the following medications at 0800: famotidine (Pepcid) 20 mg po and spironolactone (Aldactone) 50 mg po. Which action by the nurse is most appropriate?
   a. Hold the morning dose of famotidine until the physician returns the call.
   (b.) Hold the morning dose of spironolactone until the physician returns the call.
   c. Hold all the morning medications until the physician returns the call.
   d. Give all the morning medications as ordered.

Rationale: The answer is (b). Spironolactone is a potassium-sparing diuretic. Since the morning serum K^+ level is high, the drug should be held until further orders are obtained from the doctor. Option (a) does not affect the potassium level. Options (c) and (d) do not correlate the effects of the specific drugs to the laboratory work.

2. The nurse is caring for a client with diabetes mellitus type 2. The following medications are listed on the client's medication record: metformin (Glucophage) 0.5 g po bid and repaglinide (Prandil) 1 mg po with meals. The morning blood glucose fingerstick is 98 mg/dl. Which action by the nurse is most appropriate?
   a. Hold the morning po medications.
   b. Give the metformin but hold the repaglinide.
   c. Give the repaglinide but hold the metformin.
   (d.) Give the po medications as ordered.

Rationale: The answer is (d). The morning fingerstick result is within normal limits. Drug therapy should continue as ordered to maintain the blood glucose within normal limits. Options (a), (b), and (c) would not help the client remain in glycemic control.

3. The client with end-stage renal disease is scheduled for hemodialysis in 2 hours. He has a (L) AV fistula and needs assistance with feeding. In delegating the care of the client, which nursing order is of priority?
   a. Feed the client first.
   b. Give all morning care before the dialysis.
   (c.) Take the blood pressure in the right arm.
   d. Feel for a vibration on the left arm.

Rationale: The answer is (c). The AV fistula is the vascular access for the hemodialysis. Care must be taken not to occlude or cause trauma to the site. Options (a) and (b) are important but not the priority nursing order. Option (d) is part of the assessment process that is the responsibility of the professional nurse.

APPLYING CRITICAL THINKING SKILLS TO TEST QUESTIONS

INSTRUCTIONS: Circle the best answer for each test question. Write your rationale for selecting the answer. To enhance your learning and test-taking skills, discuss your answer and rationale with a partner. The answer and the rationale can be found on the back of this page.

1. At 10:00 AM the nurse realizes that clonidine (Catapres) 0.1 mg po was administered to the wrong client at 9:00 AM. Which nursing action is of priority?
   a. Fill out an incident report.
   b. Notify the physician.
   c. Take the client's blood pressure.
   d. Take the vital signs of the client at noon.

Rationale: ____________________

2. A beta-blocking agent is added to the pharmacologic therapy of a client with congestive heart failure. An expected therapeutic effect is:
   a. a decrease in complaints of fatigue.
   b. a decrease in the heart rate.
   c. an increase in blood pressure.
   d. an increase in diuresis.

Rationale: ____________________

3. The client is taking hydrochorothiazide (Esedrix) 25 mg po daily and is started on the ACE inhibitor lisinopril (Zestril) 10 mg po daily. Which nursing intervention indicates the most appropriate follow-through action?
   a. Monitor the client's output.
   b. Assess the client for impaired skin integrity.
   c. Assess the client's cardiac rhythm.
   d. Monitor the client's blood pressure.

Rationale: ____________________

FIVE

APPLYING CRITICAL THINKING SKILLS TO TEST QUESTIONS

HELPFUL HINTS: Read all test questions carefully. Identify key words in the question that will guide you in answering the question. In these test questions the **key words** to consider are **"priority," "expected therapeutic effect,"** and **"most appropriate."** Compare your rationale with the one in the test question.

1. At 10:00 AM the nurse realizes that clonidine (Catapres) 0.1 mg po was administered to the wrong client at 9:00 AM. Which nursing action is of priority?
   a. Fill out an incident report.
   b. Notify the physician.
   (c.) Take the client's blood pressure.
   d. Take the vital signs of the client at noon.

Rationale: The answer is (c). Clonidine is an alpha-adrenergic agonist and blocking agent. After oral administration, clonidine begins to exert its effect within 1 hour. Option (a) is necessary, but assessing the client is priority. Option (b) is important, but it will be important to inform the physician of the current blood pressure. Option (d) is a good follow-up intervention but not the priority intervention.

2. A beta-blocking agent is added to the pharmacologic therapy of a client with congestive heart failure. An expected therapeutic effect is:
   a. a decrease in complaints of fatigue.
   (b.) a decrease in the heart rate.
   c. an increase in blood pressure.
   d. an increase in diuresis.

Rationale: The answer is (b). Beta-blockers have multiple cardiac uses. The physiologic effect is to decrease cardiac contractibility and workload. The client may have an increase, rather than a decrease, in fatigue after beginning therapy—option (a). Options (c) and (d) do not address the mechanism of action of beta-blockers.

3. The client is taking hydrochorothiazide (Esedrix) 25 mg po daily and is started on the ACE inhibitor lisinopril (Zestril) 10 mg po daily. Which nursing intervention indicates the most appropriate follow-through action?
   a. Monitor the client's output.
   b. Assess the client for impaired skin integrity.
   c. Assess the client's cardiac rhythm.
   (d.) Monitor the client's blood pressure.

Rationale: The answer is (d). The combination of drug therapy indicates the primary use is for the antihypertensive effects. Blood pressure should be monitored. Options (a), (b), and (c) do not address the effects of the combined drug therapy.

APPLYING CRITICAL THINKING SKILLS TO TEST QUESTIONS

INSTRUCTIONS: Circle the one best answer for each test question. Write your rationale for selecting the answer. To enhance your learning and test-taking skills, discuss your answer and rationale with a partner. The answer and the rationale can be found on the back of this page.

1. The home health nurse visits a client who has a history of congestive heart failure. The client is on enalapril (Vasotec), furosemide (Lasix), and isosorbide (Isordil). While talking with the client, the nurse notices that the client has a persistent dry, nonproductive cough. Which nursing action is most appropriate?
   a. Ask if the client is taking any cough medicine.
   b. Encourage the client to increase fluid intake.
   c. Ask if the client has had any chest pain.
   d. Notify the physician.

Rationale: ______________________________

2. The nurse is providing discharge instructions to an elderly client taking the following oral medications: wafarin (Coumadin) 5 mg daily, furosemide (Lasix) 20 mg daily, and digoxin (Lanoxin) 25 mg every other day. Which of the following is most important for the nurse to include in the instructions?
   a. "You can take the pills with meals."
   b. "Call the doctor if you notice any bruising."
   c. "Use a pill box to remind you of the medicines you need to take."
   d. "Take the furosemide in the morning so that you can sleep at night."

Rationale: ______________________________

3. The nurse is delegating the care of a stable client who had a chest tube inserted after complications with the insertion of a central subclavian line the night before. Which intervention is most important for the nurse to ask the nursing assistant to carry out?
   a. Count the respiratory rate for 1 full minute.
   b. Keep the client in a high-Fowler's position.
   c. Encourage the client to cough and deep breathe.
   d. Ask the client to remain in bed while the chest tube is in place.

Rationale: ______________________________

APPLYING CRITICAL THINKING SKILLS TO TEST QUESTIONS

HELPFUL HINTS: Read all test questions carefully. Identify key words in the question that will guide you in answering the question. In these test questions the **key words** to consider are "**most appropriate**" and "**most important.**" Compare your rationale with the one in the test question.

1. The home health nurse visits a client who has a history of congestive heart failure. The client is on enalapril (Vasotec), furosemide (Lasix), and isosorbide (Isordil). While talking with the client, the nurse notices that the client has a persistent dry, nonproductive cough. Which nursing action is most appropriate?
   a. Ask if the client is taking any cough medicine.
   b. Encourage the client to increase fluid intake.
   c. Ask if the client has had any chest pain.
   (d.) Notify the physician.

Rationale: The answer is (d). A dry, nonproductive cough is a side effect of ACE inhibitors like enalapril. This may warrant a change in therapy. Options (a), (b), and (c) do not address this side effect.

2. The nurse is providing discharge instructions to an elderly client taking the following oral medications: wafarin (Coumadin) 5 mg daily, furosemide (Lasix) 20 mg daily, and digoxin (Lanoxin) 25 mg every other day. Which of the following is most important for the nurse to include in the instructions?
   a. "You can take the pills with meals."
   (b.) "Call the doctor if you notice any bruising."
   c. "Use a pill box to remind you of the medicines you need to take."
   d. "Take the furosemide in the morning so that you can sleep at night."

Rationale: The answer is (b). Based on this situation, it is most important to teach the client to recognize signs of excessive anticoagulation therapy. Options (a) and (d) are good but not the most important. Option (c) may not be the best because mixing digoxin with the other pills may be confusing for the elderly client if the digoxin needs to be held.

3. The nurse is delegating the care of a stable client who had a chest tube inserted after complications with the insertion of a central subclavian line the night before. Which intervention is most important for the nurse to ask the nursing assistant to carry out?
   a. Count the respiratory rate for 1 full minute.
   b. Keep the client in a high-Fowler's position.
   (c.) Encourage the client to cough and deep breathe.
   d. Ask the client to remain in bed while the chest tube is in place.

Rationale: The answer is (c). Clients with chest tubes should be encouraged to cough and deep breathe to enhance lung reexpansion. Options (a) and (b) are good but not the most important. Option (d) is not appropriate, and, unless contraindicated, the client should be encouraged to ambulate.

APPLYING CRITICAL THINKING SKILLS TO TEST QUESTIONS

INSTRUCTIONS: Circle the one best answer for each test question. Write your rationale for selecting the answer. To enhance your learning and test-taking skills, discuss your answer and rationale with a partner. The answer and the rationale can be found on the back of this page.

1. The client is on a heparin infusion after being diagnosed with a venous thrombus in the right leg. To best monitor the effect of the heparin therapy, the nurse would:
   a. assess for signs and symptoms of bleeding.
   b. check the aPTT.
   c. monitor the PT.
   d. check the stool for occult blood.

Rationale: ____________________

2. The nurse is assigned to a client who is 4 days postop thoracic surgery and has a chest tube. The nurse learns in morning report that there has not been any drainage from the chest tube for the last 24 hours. In assessing the closed-chest drainage system, the nurse notes that there are no fluctuations in the water-seal chamber. The client's respirations are 22, unlabored. In planning the client care, the nurse would prepare:
   a. for possible chest tube removal.
   b. for replacement of the chest tube.
   c. to increase the suction to the drainage system.
   d. to disconnect the chest tube from the drainage system.

Rationale: ____________________

3. The nurse is caring for a client who is elderly, extremely confused, and restless this morning. The client is receiving oxygen, has a chest tube, and is continuously pulling at the tube. Which is the best plan of care for this client?
   a. Assign a staff RN to care for the client.
   b. Ask the nursing assistant to monitor the client and report changes.
   c. Assign a nursing assistant, but have the RN check the client q2h.
   d. Ask the LVN/LPN to care for the client and get an order for restraints.

Rationale: ____________________

APPLYING CRITICAL THINKING SKILLS TO TEST QUESTIONS

HELPFUL HINTS: : Read all test questions carefully. Identify key words in the question that will guide you in answering the question. In these test questions the **key words** to consider are "**best**" and "**planning the client care.**" Compare your rationale with the one in the test question.

1. The client is on a heparin infusion after being diagnosed with a venous thrombus in the right leg. To best monitor the effect of the heparin therapy, the nurse would:
   a. assess for signs and symptoms of bleeding.
   (b.) check the aPTT.
   c. monitor the PT.
   d. check the stool for occult blood.

Rationale: The answer is (b). The aPTT (activated partial thromboplastin time) is used to monitor heparin therapy. Options (a) and (d) are good nursing interventions, but signs and symptoms are not the best indicators. Option (c) is mainly used to monitor wafarin therapy.

2. The nurse is assigned to a client who is 4 days postop thoracic surgery and has a chest tube. The nurse learns in morning report that there has not been any drainage from the chest tube for the last 24 hours. In assessing the closed-chest drainage system, the nurse notes that there are no fluctuations in the water-seal chamber. The client's respirations are 22, unlabored. In planning the client care, the nurse would prepare:
   (a.) for possible chest tube removal.
   b. for replacement of the chest tube.
   c. to increase the suction to the drainage system.
   d. to disconnect the chest tube from the drainage system.

Rationale: The answer is (a). The client is 4 days postop. Respiratory signs indicate normal progression of lung reexpansion. Assessment findings do not support option (b). Options (c) and (d) demonstrate a need to review chest tubes and the drainage system.

3. The nurse is caring for a client who is elderly, extremely confused, and restless this morning. The client is receiving oxygen, has a chest tube, and is continuously pulling at the tube. Which is the best plan of care for this client?
   (a.) Assign a staff RN to care for the client.
   b. Ask the nursing assistant to monitor the client and report changes.
   c. Assign a nursing assistant, but have the RN check the client q2h.
   d. Ask the LVN/LPN to care for the client and get an order for restraints.

Rationale: The answer is (a). Clients whose medical condition is unstable should be assigned to the RN. The RN is the most appropriate person to assess and monitor for changes. Options (b) and (c) are not appropriate for this client who is medically unstable. Option (d) is not the best plan.

APPLYING CRITICAL THINKING SKILLS TO TEST QUESTIONS

INSTRUCTIONS: Circle the one best answer for each test question. Write your rationale for selecting the answer. To enhance your learning and test-taking skills, discuss your answer and rationale with a partner. The answer and the rationale can be found on the back of this page.

1. The client is being treated with continuous heparin infusion for a pulmonary embolus. The morning result of the activated partial thromboplastin time (aPTT) is 100 sec (control 30 sec). Which nursing intervention is of priority?
   a. Continue to monitor the client.
   b. Take the client's vital signs.
   c. Notify the physician.
   d. Check the previous result.

Rationale: ______________________________

2. The nurse is caring for a client who has a chest tube connected to a closed-chest drainage system with suction. In assessing the water-seal chamber, the nurse notes constant bubbling. Which nursing intervention is most appropriate?
   a. Document the findings.
   b. Continue to monitor the client.
   c. Check the chest tube for air leaks.
   d. Decrease the amount of suction.

Rationale: ______________________________

3. The nurse is totaling the chest tube output at 1400, the close of the shift. The chest tube drainage is at the 125 mL calibrated mark on the drainage device. The vertical tape along the side of the calibrated marks of the drainage device has a line drawn at 50 mL with the time of 0600. Which nursing intervention is most appropriate on the basis of this finding?
   a. Draw a line at 125 mL and indicate 1400.
   b. Document 125 mL as the output for the shift.
   c. Assess the suction chamber for patency.
   d. Notify the charge nurse.

Rationale: ______________________________

APPLYING CRITICAL THINKING SKILLS TO TEST QUESTIONS

HELPFUL HINTS: Read all test questions carefully. Identify key words in the question that will guide you in answering the question. In these test questions the **key words** to consider are **"priority"** and **"most appropriate."** Compare your rationale with the one in the test question.

1. The client is being treated with continuous heparin infusion for a pulmonary embolus. The morning result of the activated partial thromboplastin time (aPTT) is 100 sec (control 30 sec). Which nursing intervention is of priority?
   a. Continue to monitor the client.
   b. Take the client's vital signs.
   (c.) Notify the physician.
   d. Check the previous result.

Rationale: The answer is (c). The goal of heparin infusion is to maintain the activated partial thromboplastin time at 1.5 to 2, the normal range. The 100 sec result is a critical value, and the client is at risk for bleeding. Options (a), (b), and (d) are good nursing interventions but not the priority intervention.

2. The nurse is caring for a client who has a chest tube connected to a closed-chest drainage system with suction. In assessing the water-seal chamber, the nurse notes constant bubbling. Which nursing intervention is most appropriate?
   a. Document the findings.
   b. Continue to monitor the client.
   (c.) Check the chest tube for air leaks.
   d. Decrease the amount of suction.

Rationale: The answer is (c). Constant bubbling in the water-seal chamber indicates an air leak. Options (a) and (b) are good interventions but are not the most appropriate on the basis of the situation. Option (d) does not address the water-seal chamber.

3. The nurse is totaling the chest tube output at 1400, the close of the shift. The chest tube drainage is at the 125-mL calibrated mark on the drainage device. The vertical tape along the side of the calibrated marks of the drainage device has a line drawn at 50 mL with the time of 0600. Which nursing intervention is most appropriate on the basis of this finding?
   (a.) Draw a line at 125 mL and indicate 1400.
   b. Document 125 mL as the output for the shift.
   c. Assess the suction chamber for patency.
   d. Notify the charge nurse.

Rationale: The answer is (a). The nurse monitors the chest tube drainage output by drawing a line at drainage level in the chamber at the end of the shift. Options (b), (c), and (d) are not appropriate interventions.

APPLYING CRITICAL THINKING SKILLS TO TEST QUESTIONS

INSTRUCTIONS: Circle the one best answer for each test question. Write your rationale for selecting the answer. To enhance your learning and test-taking skills, discuss your answer and rationale with a partner. The answer and the rationale can be found on the back of this page.

1. The nurse assesses the client who is 1 day postop transurethral resection of the prostate. He has not had any output from the urinary catheter for 2 hours. The client has an order for intermittent bladder irrigation. Which technique is best for the nurse to use to safely carry out this order?
   a. Irrigate with 50 mL of sterile water and aspirate an equal amount of fluid.
   b. Use clean technique and irrigate until the return is free of clots.
   c. Use sterile technique and irrigate with 50 mL of solution at a time.
   d. Start a continuous bladder irrigation and infuse 200 mL over 30 minutes.

Rationale: ______________________________

2. The client has just had a generalized tonic-clonic type seizure in bed. Which nursing intervention is of priority immediately after the seizure?
   a. Document the findings.
   b. Maintain a quiet environment.
   c. Reorient the client to the surroundings.
   d. Position the client in a side-lying position.

Rationale: ______________________________

3. The nurse is assigned to a client who is 4 days postop right hip replacement. The nurse finds the client eating breakfast, sitting comfortably in a chair with the right leg crossed over the left leg. Which nursing intervention is of priority?
   a. Assess the right hip dressing.
   b. Assess the client's pain level.
   c. Check the quality of the pedal pulses of both feet.
   d. Instruct the client to keep both feet flat on the floor.

Rationale: ______________________________

APPLYING CRITICAL THINKING SKILLS TO TEST QUESTIONS

HELPFUL HINTS: Read all test questions carefully. Identify key words in the question that will guide you in answering the question. In these test questions the **key words** to consider are "**best**" and "**priority.**" Compare your rationale with the one in the test question.

1. The nurse assesses the client who is 1 day postop transurethral resection of the prostate. He has not had any output from the urinary catheter for 2 hours. The client has an order for intermittent bladder irrigation. Which technique is best for the nurse to use to safely carry out this order?
   a. Irrigate with 50 mL of sterile water and aspirate an equal amount of fluid.
   b. Use clean technique and irrigate until the return is free of clots.
   (c.) Use sterile technique and irrigate with 50 mL of solution at a time.
   d. Start a continuous bladder irrigation and infuse 200 mL over 30 minutes.

Rationale: The answer is (c). Bladder irrigation is always performed with sterile technique. Solution is gently introduced into the bladder during irrigation. Options (a), (b), and (d) do not describe how to safely and correctly carry out this technique.

2. The client has just had a generalized tonic-clonic type seizure in bed. Which nursing intervention is of priority immediately after the seizure?
   a. Document the findings.
   b. Maintain a quiet environment.
   c. Reorient the client to the surroundings.
   (d.) Position the client in a side-lying position.

Rationale: The answer is (d). Aspiration is a concern after the seizure because the client will be lethargic and oral secretions will need to be suctioned and allowed to drain. Options (a), (b), and (c) are good interventions but are not priority.

3. The nurse is assigned to a client who is 4 days postop right hip replacement. The nurse finds the client eating breakfast, sitting comfortably in a chair with the right leg crossed over the left leg. Which nursing intervention is of priority?
   a. Assess the right hip dressing.
   b. Assess the client's pain level.
   c. Check the quality of the pedal pulses of both feet.
   (d.) Instruct the client to keep both feet flat on the floor.

Rationale: The answer is (d). Crossing of the feet or legs after hip replacement may put undue tension on the operative hip and increase the risk of hip dislocation. Options (a), (b), and (c) are good interventions but are not priority.

APPLYING CRITICAL THINKING SKILLS TO TEST QUESTIONS

INSTRUCTIONS: Circle the one best answer for each test question. Write your rationale for selecting the answer. To enhance your learning and test-taking skills, discuss your answer and rationale with a partner. The answer and the rationale can be found on the back of this page.

1. The client is 4 days postop colon resection and has an NG tube to low continuous suction. The client tells the nurse that he is feeling nauseated and then vomits 100 mL of yellow-green drainage. The nurse's initial action is to:
   a. assess tube placement.
   b. administer an antiemetic.
   c. pull out the NG tube.
   d. increase the NG tube suction to moderate.

Rationale: ______________________________

____

____

____

____

2. The client has been on full-strength formula tube feeding at 60 mL/hr through the NG tube for 2 days. In delegating the care of the client, which directive, given to the nursing assistant, most indicates that the nurse is monitoring for tube feeding complications?
   a. "Let me know if the client has liquid bowel movements this shift."
   b. "Weigh the client on the stand-up scale as soon as report is over."
   c. "The client can sit in a chair for 30 minutes this morning."
   d. "Take the vital signs every 4 hours."

Rationale: ______________________________

____

____

____

____

3. The physician orders to start continuous tube feedings at 50 mL/hr. After starting the tube feeding, it is most important for the nurse to initially plan to:
   a. assess bowel sounds every shift.
   b. take the vital signs q4h.
   c. monitor residual q4h.
   d. monitor the intake and output.

Rationale: ______________________________

____

____

____

____

APPLYING CRITICAL THINKING SKILLS TO TEST QUESTIONS

HELPFUL HINTS: Read all test questions carefully. Identify key words in the question that will guide you in answering the question. In these test questions the **key words** to consider are **"initial," "most indicates,"** and **"most important."** Compare your rationale with the one in the test question.

1. The client is 4 days postop colon resection and has an NG tube to low continuous suction. The client tells the nurse that he is feeling nauseated and then vomits 100 mL of yellow-green drainage. The nurse's initial action is to:
   (a.) assess tube placement.
   b. administer an antiemetic.
   c. pull out the NG tube.
   d. increase the NG tube suction to moderate.

Rationale: The answer is (a). It is important to initially check the placement of the NG tube to ensure that the tube and suction are working. Option (b) may be performed if the nausea and vomiting do not subside. Options (c) and (d) do not help to solve the problem.

2. The client has been on full-strength formula tube feeding at 60 mL/hr through the NG tube for 2 days. In delegating the care of the client, which directive, given to the nursing assistant, most indicates that the nurse is monitoring for tube feeding complications?
   (a.) "Let me know if the client has liquid bowel movements this shift."
   b. "Weigh the client on the stand-up scale as soon as report is over."
   c. "The client can sit in a chair for 30 minutes this morning."
   d. "Take the vital signs every 4 hours."

Rationale: The answer is (a). Enteral feeding formulas can cause diarrhea. Option (b) helps to identify whether the client is gaining weight. Options (c) and (d) are directives that promote good nursing care, but they are not directly related to identifying formula complications.

3. The physician orders to start continuous tube feedings at 50 mL/hr. After starting the tube feeding, it is most important for the nurse to initially plan to
   a. assess bowel sounds every shift.
   b. take the vital signs q4h.
   (c.) monitor residual q4h.
   d. monitor the intake and output.

Rationale: The answer is (c). Residual should be checked to ensure that the client is tolerating the tube feeding. Options (a), (b), and (d) are important but are not the most important.

Section Six - Quality Nursing Practice

QUALITY NURSING PRACTICE SITUATION #1

Nursing Care Plan			
Lab/diagnostic tests	**Medications**		
ECG ☑	Ketorolac 10 mg IM q6h × 24 hr Tylenol #3 tab i po q3h prn pain Promethazine 25 mg IM q4h prn N/V Indwelling urinary catheter	VS q4h Antiembolic stockings Seq. compression device	Diet: Clear liquid - DAT Ambulate with assistance Incentive spirometer q2h
IV Fluids: 1 L lactated Ringer's q8h			
Name: CJ	Age: 60 Full code	Dx: Prostate cancer Surg: da Vinci laparoscopic radical prostatectomy	

Morning Report: "The patient is one day postop. He was possibly being discharged today, but he had some chest pain last night and I heard fine crackles on the right lower lung base. Bowel sounds are faint in the four quadrants. Vital signs are stable. The urinary catheter is patent, draining blood-tinged urine. Please encourage the patient to use the incentive spirometer and have him ambulate more today. An ECG was done last night. His doctor will be in sometime this morning."

Using Nursing Knowledge

- Based on the morning report and the nursing care plan, answer the following:
- List assessment priorities:

____

____

- Identify the priorities of the plan of care for the morning:

____

____

- List signs and symptoms that might indicate possible complications that the nurse should monitor and include in the plan of care:

____

____

Using Leadership Skills

- Consider the scope of practice and then determine the nursing interventions that may be delegated to the:

LVN/LPN:

____

____

____

____

____

Unlicensed personnel:

____

____

____

Evidence-based practice:

Use appropriate resources to answer the following question:
In clients who need a radical prostatectomy, is the da Vinci method the most desirable surgical intervention?

List **desired outcomes** of the da Vinci surgical method:

____

____

SIX

Review the Caring for the Whole Person diagram below. Use the boxes to:

1. Identify <u>**actual and potential**</u> concerns related to the **Social** needs of the client.
2. Identify the **Physiological** needs at discharge.
3. List **Individual Considerations** for the client on discharge.

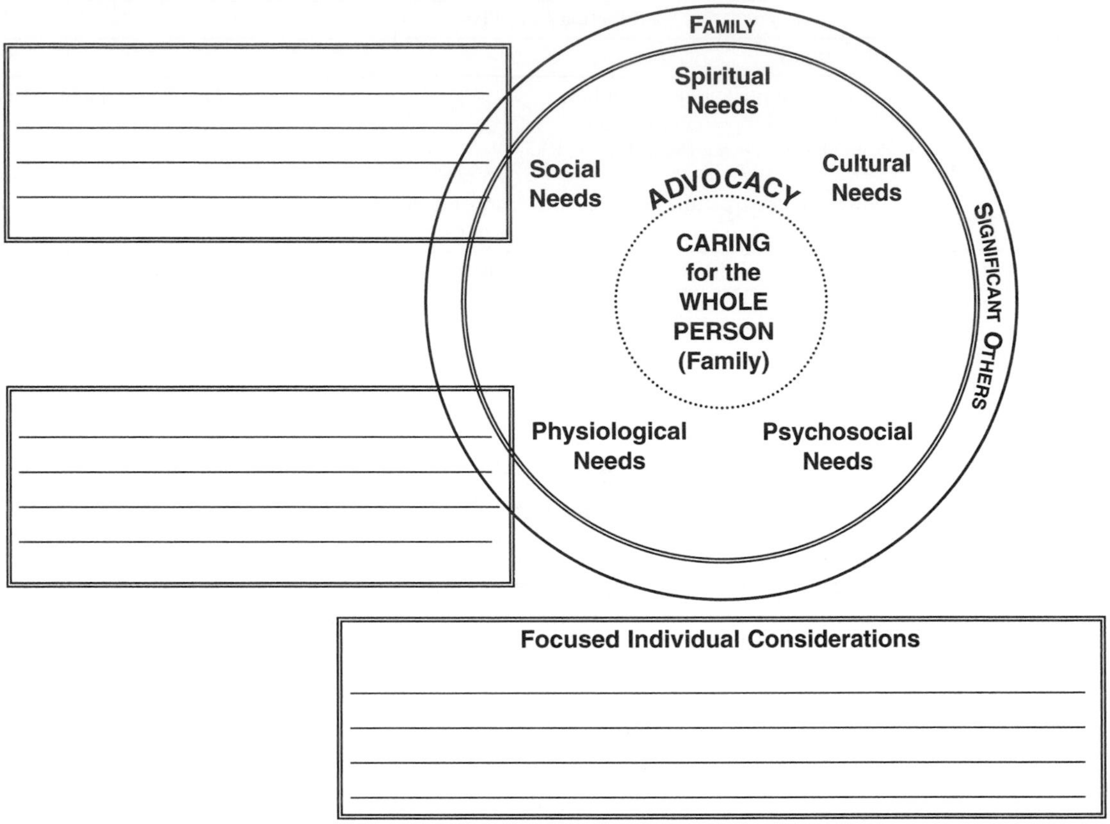

Interactive Activity: With a partner, use the textbooks and information from appropriate websites to answer and complete the possible discharge instructions for the client:

Possible discharge instructions:

Regarding urinary catheter: ______________________

Discharge medications ______________________

Activity: ______________________

Follow-up visit: ______________________

Potential complications: ______________________

QUALITY NURSING PRACTICE SITUATION #2

Nursing Care Plan		
Lab/diagnostic tests	**Medications**	
FBG in AM Electrolyte panel in AM	Lorazepam 0.5 mg IV stat	Diet: Mech soft NPO $\bar{p}$ midnight VS q4h I & O qshift Bed rest
IV fluids: 1 L Normal Saline 0.9% at 50 mL/hr		
Name: SP Age: 75	Full code	Dx: Acute confusion

Evening Report at 2300: "The client was admitted from the emergency room around 1900. The wife says that she noticed that her husband started to get confused last evening. The wife, who is 70 yrs old, has been with him all day and looks very tired. She is waiting for her son to pick her up but does not really want to leave her husband. She says they have been married 50 years and they rarely have been separated from each other. The admitting orders are on the chart. I gave him lorazepam IV for restlessness at 2100. The wife says he has been taking zolpidem for sleep. You might want to call the doctor for an order of zolpidem if the lorazepam does not calm him down."

Using Nursing Knowledge

- Based on the evening report and the nursing care plan, answer the following:
- List assessment priorities:

- Identify the priorities of the plan of care for the morning:

- List signs and symptoms that might indicate possible complications that the nurse should monitor and include in the plan of care:

Using Leadership Skills

- Consider the scope of practice, then determine the nursing interventions that may be delegated for this client to the:

LVN/LPN:

Unlicensed personnel:

Evidence-based practice:

Use appropriate resources to answer the following question:
In elderly clients using zolpidem, is confusion a common adverse effect?

List **desired outcomes** of zolpidem therapy:

SIX

Review the Caring for the Whole Person diagram below. Use the boxes to:

1. Identify <u>**actual and potential**</u> **Physiological** needs related to the care of the client.
2. Identify the <u>**actual or potential**</u> **Psychosocial** needs expressed by the <u>**wife**</u>.
3. List **Individual Considerations** for the care of the client.

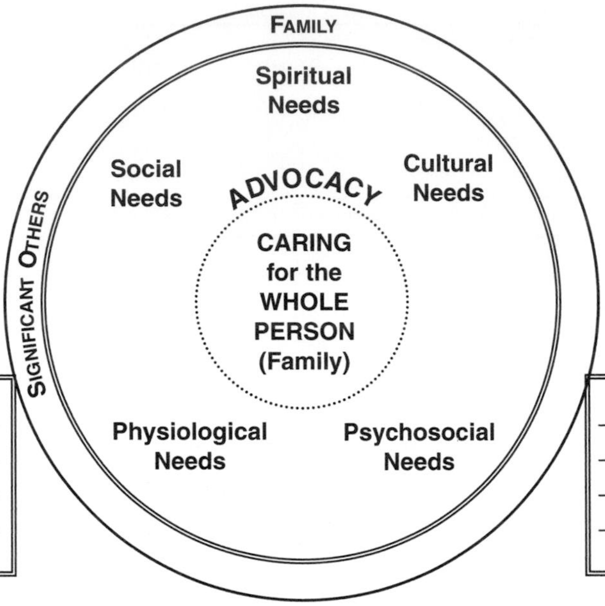

____

____

____

____

Focused Individual Considerations

____

____

____

____

Interactive Activity: With a partner, use the following part of the case scenario to write possible therapeutic communication statements that demonstrate caring and advocacy:

The wife, who is 70 yrs old, has been with him all day and looks very tired. She is waiting for her son to pick her up but does not really want to leave her husband. She says they have been married 50 years and they rarely have been separated from each other.

Write possible therapeutic communication statements that demonstrate **caring**:

1. ______________________

2. ______________________

3. ______________________

4. ______________________

Write a possible therapeutic communication statement that demonstrates **advocacy**:

____

QUALITY NURSING PRACTICE SITUATION #3

Nursing Care Plan		
	Medications	
FSBG qAM & qPM (Call MD if greater than 150 mg/dl) O_2 per N/C @ 3 L prn	Amiodipine 5 mg po daily Cimetidine 400 mg po QID Avandia 4 mg po daily Nitroglycerin 0.4 mg SL i tab q5min ×3 prn chest pain	Diet: 1800 ADA VS q4h I & O Up in chair tid Antiembolic hose
	Saline lock flush with NS qshift	
Name: RA Age: 60	Full code	Dx: Pneumonia, hypertension Hx of CAD, Unstable angina DM Type 2

Report at 0700: "The client had a restful night. He says he is going home this morning. His lungs are clear and the vital signs are stable with a BP of 140/88. He complained of some indigestion a little while ago, so I gave the cimetidine early. Aside from his routine medications and removal of his saline lock on discharge, he is ready to go."

Progression of Sentinel Event

- After report the RN visits the client and asks the client whether the cimetidine has helped him. The client says it was just given to him so that it will take a few more minutes for the drug to work. He asks for the emesis basin "just in case."
- The RN asks the unlicensed assistant to take the pulse and BP since the client is diaphoretic. Dynamap readings indicate an increase in pulse and a BP of 120/70.
- The RN asks the LVN to start the oxygen and asks the CNA to take vital signs q5min.
- The RN goes to call the physician.
- Ten minutes later the LVN calls a code. After 30 minutes of CPR the client is pronounced dead.

Using Leadership Skills

List the current needs that are associated with the care of the family experiencing the death of a loved one:

- Prepare for family visit (Who should be involved?)

____

- Postdeath care can be done by:

____

- Notify pastoral care (Who should notify?)

____

- Document (Who should document?)

____

Evaluate the situation

What could have been done differently?

____

____

Evidence-based practice:

Use appropriate resources to answer the following question:
How frequently are Rapid Response Teams used in the clinical setting?

List **desired outcomes** of using experienced staff/Rapid Response Teams:

____

____

____

Review the Caring for the Whole Person diagram below. Use the boxes to:

1. Identify **actual and potential** Psychosocial Needs for the **family** related to the unexpected death of the client.
2. List **Individual Considerations** for the postdeath care of the client.

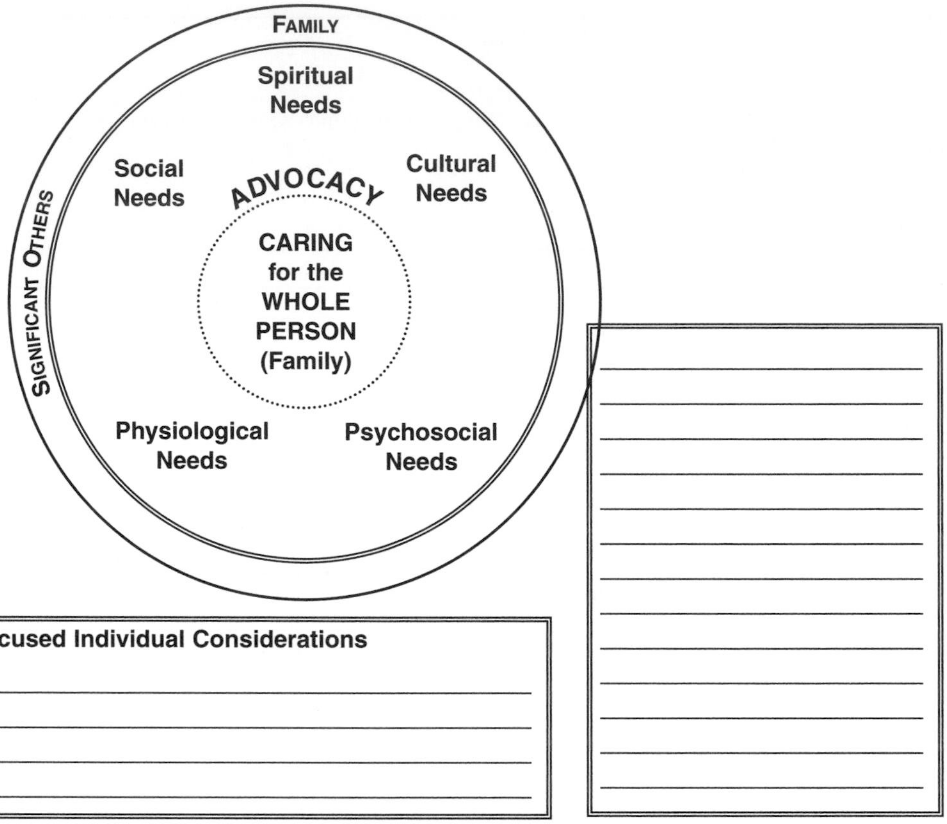

Focused Individual Considerations

____
____
____
____

Interactive Activity: With a partner, reread the situation. Discuss and answer the following:

- If you are the **staff nurse**, what could have been done differently?

____
____

- If you are the **staff nurse**, what would be most helpful now after reviewing and experiencing the sentinel event?

____
____

- If you are the **unit supervisor**, what could have been done differently?

____
____

- If you are the **unit supervisor**, what would be most helpful for the staff nurse? Unit? Hospital?

____
____

Bibliography

Ackley, B. J., & Ladwig, G. (2008). *Nursing Diagnosis Handbook.* (8th ed.) St. Louis: Mosby.

Burkhardt, M. A., & Nathaniel, A. K. (2008). *Ethics & Issues in Contemporary Nursing.* Clifton Park, New York: Thomson Delmar Learning

Deglin, J. H., & Vallerand, A. H. (2007). *Davis's Drug Guide.* (10th ed.) Philadelphia: F.A. Davis.

Harkreader, H., & Hogan, M. A. (2007). *Fundamentals of Nursing: Caring and Clinical Judgment.* (3rd ed.) St. Louis: W.B. Saunders.

Institute for Healthcare Improvement (2005). SBAR technique for communication: A situational briefing model. Retrieved May 17, 2008, from website: http://www.ihi.org

Lilley, L., Harrington, S., & Snyder, J. S. (2007). *Pharmacology and the Nursing Process.* (5th ed.) St. Louis: Mosby.

Monahan, F., Sands, J. K., Neighbors, M., Marek, J. F., & Green, C. J. (2007). *Phipps' Medical-Surgical Nursing.* (8th ed.) St. Louis: Mosby.

National Pressure Ulcer Advisory Panel (2007). Pressure ulcer stages revised by NPUAP. Retrieved May 27, 2008, from website: http://www.npuap.org

Pagana, K., & Pagana, T. (2006). *Mosby's Manual of Diagnostic and Laboratory Tests.* (3rd ed.) St. Louis: Mosby.

Seventh Report of the Joint National Committee on Prevention, Detection, Evaluation, and Treatment of High Blood Pressure (JNR7). NIH Publication No. 03-6231 May 2003, Retrieved June 17, 2008 from website: http://www.nhlbi.nih.gov/guidelines /hypertension/phycard.pdf

Ufema, J. (2007). *Insights on Death & Dying.* Philadelphia: Lippincott Williams & Wilkins

Venes, D. (2005) *Taber's Cyclopedic Medical Dictionary.* Philadelphia: F.A. Davis.

Appendix A

List of Abbreviations

ac	=	before meals
BUN	=	blood urea nitrogen
BM	=	bowel movement
BR	=	bedrest
Client	=	patient
CBC	=	complete blood count
Dx	=	diagnosis
ECG	=	electrocardiogram
FBG	=	fasting blood glucose
I & O	=	intake and output
Kardex	=	Rand
NP	=	nasal prongs (same as nasal cannula = NC)
N/V	=	nausea/vomiting
NPO	=	nothing by mouth
OGTT	=	oral glucose tolerance test
PCA	=	patient-controlled analgesia
PT	=	protime
UA	=	urinalysis
VS	=	vital signs (T - P - R - BP)

T	=	temperature
P	=	pulse
R	=	respirations
BP	=	blood pressure

OOB	=	out of bed
ROM	=	range of motion

↑ Increased

↓ Decreased

> greater than
< less than

Appendix B

List of Words and Phrases Commonly Used in the Book and Their Intended Meanings

Assessment finding	=	presenting sign, symptom, laboratory data, complaint *Example:* Which assessment finding is of most concern?
Document the findings	=	to chart assessment data in the client's chart or to enter the assessment data in the computer program
Expected findings	=	assessment findings/lab data that are associated with the illness or diagnosis *Example:* A client has a hay fever allergy. ***Expected findings:*** watery, itchy eyes, clear mucus, sneezing *Example:* A client has anemia. ***Expected findings:*** decreased hemoglobin and hematocrit; serum Hgb and Hct below the normal range
Expected outcome	=	the desired outcome based on the implementation of appropriate interventions
Focused assessment	=	the signs and symptoms associated with the medical diagnosis or with the acute illness/condition
Of priority	=	the sign/symptom/intervention that is of most concern *Example:* Which intervention is of priority . . .
Most effective	=	most appropriate for the situation *Example:* The most effective infection control method . . .
To effectively	=	to appropriately *Example:* To effectively use the incentive spirometer . . .
To implement	=	to put into action; to carry out *Example:* To implement this order effectively . . .
Predisposed	=	at risk or likely to develop *Example:* A client who smokes is predisposed to developing adverse lung conditions
The primary purpose	=	the most important reason or the primary reason *Example:* The primary purpose of the . . .

The Joint Commission

Official "Do Not Use" List[1]

Do Not Use	Potential Problem	Use Instead
U (unit)	Mistaken for "0" (zero), the number "4" (four) or "cc"	Write "unit"
IU (International Unit)	Mistaken for IV (intravenous) or the number 10 (ten)	Write "International Unit"
Q.D., QD, q.d., qd (daily) Q.O.D., QOD, q.o.d, qod (every other day)	Mistaken for each other Period after the Q mistaken for "I" and the "O" mistaken for "I"	Write "daily" Write "every other day"
Trailing zero (X.0 mg)* Lack of leading zero (.X mg)	Decimal point is missed	Write X mg Write 0.X mg
MS MSO_4 AND $MgSO_4$	Can mean morphine sulfate or magnesium sulfate Confused for one another	Write "morphine sulfate" Write "magnesium sulfate"

[1]Applies to all orders and all medication-related documentation that is handwritten (including free-text computer entry) or on pre-printed forms.

***Exception:** A "trailing zero" may be used only where required to demonstrate the level of precision of the value being reported, such as for laboratory results, imaging studies that report size of lesions, or catheter/tube sizes. It may not be used in medication orders or other medication-related documentation.

Additional Abbreviations, Acronyms and Symbols

(For possible future inclusion in the Official "Do Not Use" List)

Do Not Use	Potential Problem	Use Instead
> (greater than) < (less than)	Misinterpreted as the number "7" (seven) or the letter "L" Confused for one another	Write "greater than" Write "less than"
Abbreviations for drug names	Misinterpreted due to similar abbreviations for multiple drugs	Write drug names in full
Apothecary units	Unfamiliar to many practitioners Confused with metric units	Use metric units
@	Mistaken for the number "2" (two)	Write "at"
cc	Mistaken for U (units) when poorly written	Write "ml" or "milliliters"
μg	Mistaken for mg (milligrams) resulting in one thousand-fold overdose	Write "mcg" or "micrograms"

NOTES

NOTES